WOF
COM
IN HEA
HUMA

WORKING WITH COMMUNITIES
IN HEALTH AND HUMAN SERVICES

Judy Taylor,
David Wilkinson
and Brian Cheers

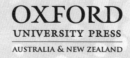

OXFORD
UNIVERSITY PRESS
AUSTRALIA & NEW ZEALAND

OXFORD
UNIVERSITY PRESS
AUSTRALIA & NEW ZEALAND

253 Normanby Road, South Melbourne, Victoria 3205, Australia

Oxford University Press is a department of the University of Oxford.
It furthers the University's objective of excellence in research,
scholarship, and education by publishing worldwide in

Oxford New York

Auckland Cape Town Dar es Salaam Hong Kong Karachi
Kuala Lumpur Madrid Melbourne Mexico City Nairobi
New Delhi Shanghai Taipei Toronto

With offices in

Argentina Austria Brazil Chile Czech Republic France Greece
Guatemala Hungary Italy Japan Poland Portugal Singapore
South Korea Switzerland Thailand Turkey Ukraine Vietnam

OXFORD is a trademark of Oxford University Press
in the UK and in certain other countries

National Library of Australia Cataloguing-in-Publication data

Taylor, Judy.
    Working with communities in health and human services.

    Bibliography.
    Includes index.

    ISBN 978 0 19 555835 7 (pbk)

    1. Community health services—Citizen participation.
    2. Human services—Citizen participation.
    I. Wilkinson, David. II. Cheers, Brian. III. Title.

362.12

Edited by Valina Rainer
Cover design, text design and typeset by Kerry Cooke, eggplant communications
Proofread by Roy Garner
Indexed by Neale Towart
Printed in Hong Kong by Sheck Wah Tong Press Ltd.

Contents

Figures, Tables, Case Examples and Activities

Figures

Tables

Case examples

Activities

Preface

We have come together from diverse perspectives—social work, medicine, public health, management, community sociology, and community development—to write this book because we believe that multiple levels of action—individual, organisational, and community—are necessary if we are to improve health and wellbeing. As practitioners, we are aware that the rhetoric about the importance of engaging communities and building community capacity is not always matched with resources and information that would support this happening. The reorientation of governments and organisations towards a greater focus on working with communities has resulted in a need for a new set of skills.

The book argues that communities can and do become involved in effective health and social care development—they initiate, plan for, implement, monitor, and evaluate neighbourhood centres, Aboriginal Community Controlled Health Services, accommodation services, men's health centres, and much more. However, we also acknowledge that these activities will be most effective if health and human service professionals and governments at all levels work together. The book provides both a theoretical base and a practice framework to enable these partnerships to flourish. The information can be applied across the spectrum of health and human services, and the conceptual framework used is underpinned by our current and recent research.

Our practice in service development in urban, rural, remote, and regional locations in Australia, the United Kingdom, Canada, and South Africa provides a foundation for writing the book. In addition, our community research has helped clarify the principles that underpin effective work with communities, the different approaches that are taken, and the community capacities that are related to good outcomes. Specific research has been conducted to prepare case studies that illustrate the issues.

The book is useful for undergraduate students and also practitioners in the fields of social work, primary health care, allied health, community work, youth work, and social planning. It is also valuable for community members and local government, and it is not discipline-specific.

Working to develop community-based health and human services can be a very rewarding experience. It may result in getting to know people who will introduce you to different ways of understanding the world and who have localised and in-depth knowledge about community wellbeing and how to work towards it. Programs that you have helped developed may, over long periods of time, add significantly to community development and sustainability. Health services, employment programs and housing co-ops are an important part of the social infrastructure in urban, rural, remote, and regional locations. Communities of all types express themselves through developing services and initiatives.

Communities of place and communities of interest

We discuss working to develop health and wellbeing with 'communities of place' and 'communities of interest'. 'A community of place is characterised by three components: locality, local society and a process of locality-oriented collective actions' (Cheers 2001, p. 130). Most rural and remote localities in Australia are 'communities of place', but also localities in cities and regional centres can be understood in this way.

'Communities of place' may also include 'communities of interest'. We define the latter, from the work of Guterbock (1990, p. 92) as: 'groups of people where there are interactions and a degree of integration because of economic, social, political and/or cultural connections and similarities between people'.

This book is for communities too

Recent information about working with communities is almost always from the perspective of professionals; those people employed in health or human services whose task it is to 'engage' with communities in health promotion, or 'build their capacity' to solve social development problems. It has not been from the perspective of the communities involved. We argue, from our research, that communities may see things differently. They may see participation to achieve a specific task but more broadly related to the betterment of the community. Therefore, we focus both on community perspectives and perspectives of the people who work with communities in developing services or programs. The book provides information that may enable effective negotiation of the conflicts that inevitably arise because of these divergent perspectives.

The plan of the book

The book is divided into three parts, dealing respectively with:

➤ theory and concepts used to understand communities;
➤ conceptual approaches to and practice frameworks for working with communities; and
➤ practical skills in working with communities.

Part 1: Understanding communities

Chapter 1 presents a definition of community health and social care development, and the two key principles in working with communities. The principles are that community work involves relationships and partnerships, and an in-depth understanding of communities. It is through a shared understanding of the community and purposive working relationships that changes that will benefit the health and wellbeing of community members occur.

Theory and concepts helpful in understanding different types of communities as a prelude to working with them are introduced in Chapter 2. Two theoretical approaches are presented. Community interaction theory developed by Wilkinson (1991) and Sharp (2001) from social field theory (Kaufman 1959; Wilkinson 1970) is used to explore community structures, elements and processes that generate improved capacity for community action. The concept of a community as a multidimensional system (Walter 2005), evident in current approaches to community-based health promotion, is also presented.

In Chapter 3, we explore some Australian Aboriginal understandings of community, which are different from Western understandings. We do this through dialogues with Rachael Cummins, Ian Gentle, and Charmaine Hull.

Chapter 4 is about community capacity, and includes contemporary definitions and ways of assessing it.

Part 2: Approaches to working with communities

Part 2 focuses on the approaches and frameworks used in policy and practice to work with communities in developing community health and social wellbeing.

Chapter 5 constructs a typology of contemporary conceptual approaches to working with communities, as the 'contributions', the 'instrumental', the 'community empowerment', and the 'developmental' approaches.

Chapter 6 presents five practice frameworks from community development and health promotion practice to illustrate the steps involved in community health and social care development.

Chapter 7 demonstrates two government approaches to working with communities: community services development (CSD) and community engagement.

Part 3: Skills in working with communities

Part 3 presents information about the skills involved in working with communities. The skill sets are presented as interrelated and generic across all disciplines and useful for both practitioners and community members. Each of the chapters outlines one of the sets of skills, identified by the aspect of working with communities to which it relates:

➤ Chapter 8, community decision-making;
➤ Chapter 9, building and maintaining community partnerships;
➤ Chapter 10, community leadership;
➤ Chapter 11, community planning; and
➤ Chapter 12, building knowledge about community health and social care development.

Using the activities and case examples

Each chapter has a number of activities and case examples that have been designed especially to illustrate the points being made in the text. The case examples and activities are drawn from community health and social care practice. Where the source of a case example or activity is acknowledged, it is a real-life example. If a source is not acknowledged, then the example is fictitious. All of the case examples and activities are intended to reflect the general principles involved in working with communities rather than a particular discipline's approach to the situation. We believe that the use of case examples and activities best illustrates the principles, approaches, and issues in working with communities.

We suggest doing activities as group activities, as group discussion can best illustrate the different ways to practise. It will become apparent that there is no 'one right way', and that people's approaches will be influenced by their discipline, their values and experiences. By integrating people's experiences with the concepts and practical skills presented in this book, they will be of most value in learning about working with communities.

The practice tips included throughout the book can be used as reminders of key components of particular activities, for example, setting up a community advisory committee. Websites are listed at the end of each chapter and provide practical information about the topics discussed in the chapter.

Acknowledgments

The process of authors bringing together diverse perspectives across disciplines has been stimulating and rewarding. So, many thanks to the co-authors. Sonia Champion did the painting on the cover, using traditional Aboriginal symbolism to reflect working with communities, and we are privileged to have her contribution. Also sincere thanks to our publisher, Debra James, who believed in the content and has been a wise adviser.

Long and vigorous debates in coffee shops, under mango trees, in single-engine planes, restaurants, planning meetings, motels, and four-wheel drives with my Queensland colleagues, including Viv Atkinson, Majella Ryan, Ros Hayes, Jan Williams, Tricia Hays, Jill Wilson, Tim Gleeson, David James, and Maurie O'Connor, helped develop the concepts on which this book is built.

Then there are those many people who work for their communities who have contributed immeasurably to this work, including Ian Gentle, Charmaine Hull, Rachel Cummins, Robyrta Felton, Hillyer Johnnie, Joan Heatley, Julie Walder, Truffy Maginnis, Ric Thomson, Val Brodie, and Peter Kelly.

More recently, my colleagues at the Spencer Gulf Rural Health School and the Primary Health Care Research Evaluation and Development program, particularly Dianne Fraser, have supported the work. But it is family and friends that really made it possible for this book to see the light of day, and I am indebted to them all—especially Jane.

Judy Taylor

Case studies were kindly provided by:
Bfriend, UnitingCare Wesley, Adelaide, SA
Sera's Women's Shelter, Townsville, NQ
Panthers on the Prowl Community Development Foundation, Penrith, NSW
In Our Hands Health Centre, Whyalla, SA
Community and Cultural Services Consultancy Unit, Townsville City Council, NQ

Robyrta Felton, Hillyer Johnnie, and Marlene Speechley, NQ
Pika Wiya Health Service, Port Augusta, SA
Pauline Zanet, Spencer Gulf Rural Health School, Whyalla Norrie, SA
Frances Parker and colleagues, University of Western Sydney, NSW
Jo McLeay, Jillian Parker, and members of the Burning Issues Exhibition Committee, Eyre Peninsula, SA
Lib Hylton Keele, Department of Primary Industries and Resources, SA

PART 1

Understanding Communities

Chapter 1 introduces community health and social care development, and justifies why they are important in the contemporary context.

Chapter 2 provides theory and concepts to understand 'community', and examines communities of place, communities of interest, and communities as a social system.

Chapter 3 explores three perspectives on what the term 'community' means to Aboriginal Australians, and this chapter is written as interviews with Rachel Cummins, Ian Gentle, and Charmaine Hull.

Chapter 4 introduces the concept of community capacity, and describes several approaches to measurement and capacity-building.

CHAPTER 1

Community Health and Social Care Development

Introduction

This chapter will:

➤ define how the terms 'community health development' and 'social care development' are used in this book;

➤ explain why the principle of community involvement underpins most community health and social care development;

➤ explain why it is important to understand the 'community' that is to be involved in this work;

➤ explain the reasons why partnerships between communities, practitioners, organisations, governments, and funding agencies are fundamental in community health and social care development.

What is community health and social care development?

'Community health development' and 'social care development' are the terms used throughout this book to refer to 'communities working together with practitioners and governments to assess social and health needs and issues, and organise and implement effective strategies to meet those needs' (Zakus and Lysack 1998, p. 2). The processes involved in working in community health and social care development are similar, and the outcomes are often interrelated. For example, an exercise program to encourage a healthy lifestyle may have social benefits for participants, such as making new friends.

The practice of community health and social care development is not discipline-specific, and a range of personnel may be engaged in working together. Social workers at neighbourhood centres, Lifeline volunteers, a leisure centre providing men's health programs, or a manager of a charitable trust may all be involved in developing health and social care services and programs. Because of the range of activities that can be legitimately called community health and social care development, it is important that we define how we are using these terms.

Defining social care and community health

'Social care' is defined as those arrangements within society, other than the market, that have the primary function of providing for the material, social, and emotional wellbeing and development of citizens (Cheers et al. 2007). In Australia, practitioners have an assortment of professional backgrounds and qualifications, primarily in social work, nursing, human services, education, and psychology, and work in a variety of fields, such as family welfare, community development, education, youth work, corrections, and health.

Human services, such as child care, counselling and crisis accommodation services, and services provided through neighbourhood centres, are all part of social care provision. Social care also includes everyday activities, such as someone helping look after a neighbour's children when the parent goes to a doctor's appointment or farmers helping each other out with fencing properties after a bushfire.

'Community health' is a term used in population health, public health, and primary health care to describe the setting where interventions to prevent disease and improve health take place. McMurray (1999, p. 7) defines 'community health' as a 'synthesis of healthy people and healthy environments'. It includes the provision of all types of community-based health care, but also the maintenance of a clean and safe environment, public policy that supports healthy lifestyles, health promotion, and primary prevention. Primary prevention is the activities and interventions designed to keep people well, before there are any manifestations of illness. Examples include immunisation programs and programs to encourage healthy eating. Disciplines involved in developing community health include nursing, medicine, public health, social work, and health administration.

Community health development involves planning processes to identify health needs and priorities, making decisions about how those needs will be met, and implementing and evaluating programs and services to meet those needs. It may also involve highlighting the health benefits of activities that occur naturally, such as exercising through walking with friends, and encouraging others to do so. The processes involved in social care development are similar, including identifying social issues with communities and deciding how these issues will be addressed, either through establishing and maintaining community services or strengthening social relationships, or both. Community health and social care development always involves partnerships between communities, practitioners, government, and non-government agencies.

Why work with communities?

> Because of the problems we have with housing, with unemployment, and with our kids getting into trouble—all these issues we talk about—they are all stressful and it is sort of like one big circle, isn't it? We go back and back to the same problems that affect everything. (Community member at a health planning session)

It is well accepted that working in partnership with communities in the places where people live is important because it is here that we can most directly take into account the social and economic factors that affect health and wellbeing, address health inequalities between groups, and help build high-quality relevant programs and initiatives (Labonte 2005). From the practitioner's perspective, working at the community level offers significant opportunities to engage with whole communities in planning to address health and wellbeing issues in a way that includes marginalised groups and considers the contextual issues that will impact on the program or services. It is not a 'one size fits all' approach, and has the added advantage of building relationships at the community level.

Second, communities that can respond to their needs and develop programs and services that benefit the community as a whole demonstrate community capacity and community strength. Cheers (1999, p. 2) describes this well when he talks about the role that human services traditionally play in strengthening rural communities.

> In a rural community, social care arrangements provide an important forum through which people can care for their community and each other—to participate in 'community agency'. They do this by helping each other and through involvement in community organisations, volunteer work, agency management, community development, and social planning. Reduce the viability of a community's social care organisations and we diminish community agency. Diminish community agency and we weaken community.

Community involvement in the management and development of services usually results in a sense of local ownership (Cheers 1998, p. 149). Community input into planning helps ensure that programs are accountable, efficient, contextualised, and effectively targeted to local needs (Laverack 2003). Taking collective action about issues can help residents experience a connection to the community that may lead to a sense of achievement and an acknowledgment that the community is likely to be able to sustain itself into the future. This is reassuring to everyone.

Working with communities to facilitate collective action aimed at community betterment overall, in addition to health and social care benefits, is justified by the evidence that 'community' is a factor in the wellbeing of people (Wilkinson 1979) and the types of relationships we form in everyday life are a factor in determining health (Kawachi et al. 1997; Veenstra 2000; Veenstra et al. 2005). Therefore, we have two groups of reasons for working with communities in developing community health and social care. We work both to address the social determinants of health and to develop the community. Generally, these aspects go hand-in-hand and they are interrelated and inseparable (Hawe et al. 1997, p. 34).

Here is an example that illustrates how developing the community and addressing health and social care issues are intertwined.

CASE EXAMPLE 1.1

Developing community, addressing health issues

Source: Zanet et al. 2005

A small community was worried about diminishing participation in the local hospital board. Because of a downturn in the agricultural industry and the economic base of the town, people were entering fulltime employment and having to travel to a regional centre. What time was left was spent with family, and people were reluctant to attend meetings to get involved in health issues. At the annual general meeting there were no nominations for the position of chairperson or secretary of the hospital board. This resulted in a community health worker calling a community meeting to discuss issues involved in getting a viable management group for the hospital. However, what people discussed at the meeting were the problems the community was facing with unemployment, young adults having to leave town, the lack of formal child care options, and the stress farmers were facing. The opportunity to voice these concerns was valued and several working groups were formed to look at what actions could be taken to address the priorities, which were seen as employment and men's health issues. Community members were aware that there were few opportunities to get together across the age ranges now that people were away from the community during the day. They thought that working together on an issue might be one way connections between community members might be enhanced.

> ## Think about it
> ➤ What are some of the social determinants of health that may affect community members in this case example?
> ➤ What are some actions that the community could take to address its issues?
> ➤ What are some of the roles the community health worker could take in working with the community?

Links between community and health and wellbeing

The social and economic factors that influence how long people live, and how well they live, are referred to as the social determinants of health. Some of these factors operate at the community level. For example, the availability of jobs in a community affects income levels, and income levels affect access to housing and health and human services, and, in turn, all of these factors affect health and wellbeing. There is a wealth of information about the links between health status and both socio-economic status and social integration.

➤ Epidemiological studies in the UK have found that socio-economic status, and in particular inequalities between different groups of people, are positively associated with national mortality rates (Wilkinson 1996).
➤ Socially supportive relationships, whether defined through social networks or social capital, have been reported to decrease suicide rates (Hassan 1994).
➤ Socially supportive relationships are also known to buffer the effects of unemployment (Gore 1978).
➤ Socially supportive relationships improve survival terms after myocardial infarction and decrease all-cause mortality (Berkman and Glass 2000).

Furthermore, early evidence from preliminary studies (Kawachi 2001) indicates that communities with higher levels of social integration have lower suicide rates, while those with higher levels of interpersonal trust, group membership, and perceived reciprocity have lower mortality and morbidity rates on a range of indicators.

There is another link between community and health and wellbeing. Social and economic inequalities arise between groups of people living in a community because of gender, race, culture, faith, sexual preference, or capability (Minkler

2005). There are factors about community functioning that contribute to these inequalities. For example, people from a different cultural background may find it more difficult to obtain housing or employment because of racial discrimination. Members of a faith community may be seen as separate from the local society, and may not be included in community events.

Addressing social determinants of health at the community level

One of the ways to address the links between community and health and wellbeing is to work at the community level with community networks and organisations to address health and social problems. Meredith Minkler and her colleagues (2005 p. 6) stress that contemporary approaches to address the social determinants of health and wellbeing continue to frame and view health and social problems, and their solutions, in individual terms. In health, they argue, it is the roles that individuals can play that are in focus in health policy and planning.

CASE EXAMPLE 1.2

Aboriginal health is not just the domain of the health care system

Source: de Costa 2001, pp. 2162–3

The need for a multifaceted approach to improve health is never more apparent than in Indigenous health. The Wakely prize essay published in *The Lancet* in 2001 reported the case of Flora, a young Aboriginal woman who lived in a remote area of Australia. Health clinic staff in the community where Flora lived tried unsuccessfully to get her to come for a colposcopy (a special examination of the cervix). After her third pregnancy, staff noticed severe dysplasia, suggesting the possibility of early cancer. Staff were keen for Flora to take advantage of the excellent medical services available to her; however, so far the services have made almost no impact on her health.

Because there are a myriad of factors that will determine Flora's health, such as material poverty, inadequate housing, and recurrent infection, the responses we make need to take into direct consideration the levels of causation. A focus on one point or one level is simply inadequate, as Flora's situation demonstrates (Wilkinson 2002).

As Rachel Cummins, Ian Gentle, and Charmaine Hull tell us in Chapter 3, we need to be aware of the broader societal-level factors that will impact on Flora's health. Flora's people have been dispossessed and have been forced to relocate far from their land, which holds their cultural and spiritual meanings. However, in Aboriginal society, in spite of dislocation, every Aboriginal person has a place, and relationships with grandmothers, uncles, aunties, mothers, sisters, and brothers are fundamental. Understanding these relationships and working with them may assist Flora to access the health care that is available. Understanding Flora's culture and experiences will show what actions might be taken in partnership that might address her health issues as well as some community-level health determinants.

Think about it

➤ What are some of the individual-level factors that are likely to affect Flora's health?

➤ What are some of the community-level factors that are likely to affect her health?

➤ What are some of the broader, societal-level factors that are likely to affect her health?

➤ What are some of the factors that might result in Flora not attending health centre appointments?

In human service provision, community-oriented practice has declined and the language of community orientation has been replaced by the language of user/carer consultation and participation—a narrower form of practice that meets strategic objectives (Turbett 2006, p. 592). In addressing social issues, it is an approach that stresses the responsibility that individuals have to participate in individualised approaches to address unemployment, homelessness, and personal wellbeing.

However, if we continue to focus only on the individual, then many of the factors that affect health and wellbeing cannot be addressed. Case example 1.2 shows the way in which influences on health and wellbeing operate at the individual, community, and the broader societal level. Many of these factors are outside the control of the individual concerned and the highly skilled and dedicated professionals who provide the most appropriate health and social care. It is only by working together at multiple levels that community health and social care development be achieved (Wilkinson 2002).

Some issues in working with communities

There is no doubt that working at a community level to address the determinants of health and socio-emotional wellbeing is complex. The most obvious problem that practitioners face is the tension that may occur between a top-down agenda from a funding agency and the bottom-up demands of communities. Very often the strategic goals and targets that are important to health and human service organisations are not always shared by the community. In almost all the work we do with communities, there are a range of government and practitioner perspectives, and community values, attitudes, needs, and priorities that must be negotiated if services and programs are to work and to be of benefit to the key stakeholders—the community. And we must remember that the key stakeholders are the community. Therefore the work is almost always political.

Then we must acknowledge that the environment in which community development occurs is shaped by a complex web of economic, political, and social forces that operate at the community, regional, national, and international levels (Cheers et al. 2007). The term 'globalisation', meaning the internationalisation of markets and information flows, is often used in an ideological sense to explain a myriad of changes at the community level, such as rationalisation of services, contracting out, and an expectation by government of communities doing things for themselves. There is no doubt that these reforms challenge communities, produce stress, and often reduce the level of control they have over their economies and service-delivery systems (Taylor 1999). On the positive side, altered circumstances may provide new openings, and it is important to work with communities to manage the changes and respond to opportunities.

The other factor that makes the work complex is that the processes involved are interrelated, and work cannot proceed in a set sequence. For example, while community involvement in planning about a project should be the first step, this is impractical when a project is being implemented through a targeting process and the community has not actually asked for the program. Therefore, forming relationships is the first step, and the processes involved in planning, decision-making, community leadership, and developing partnerships are all interwoven. The consequence of this is that it can be very difficult to know what impact your work is having and to predict what the outcomes might be.

Working with communities can be likened to trying to find a radio station on the car radio in the dark. There are lots of adjustments to the tuning, disconcerting noises, and then something comprehensible emerges, but it may not be the radio station or the program that you were looking for. So, given the difficulties inherent in working with communities, it is really important to start out with first principles.

Principles in working with communities

This section of the chapter identifies what we consider to be overarching principles in working with communities. In the following chapters, we illustrate and expand upon these principles by presenting theory, concepts, practice frameworks, and skills

The two overriding principles are:

➤ effective work with communities requires a sound understanding of the community that is being worked with; and

➤ establishing and maintaining effective working partnerships with those who are critical to the development effort is essential.

This case example illustrates these two principles.

CASE EXAMPLE 1.3

Whiteleaf: Building a healthier community

A community worker with a regional health service was allocated the task to get a community-based planning process in place to make the town eligible for a funding from a government health initiative aimed at primary prevention. Whiteleaf was one of five locations targeted because of relatively poor health service infrastructure and a difficulty in attracting a medical and allied health workforce. Government funding was to be made available to each targeted area if residents could submit a proposal to implement the project through building partnerships across the health, education, and business sectors. The regional health service, the government-funded provider of the range of acute and primary health care services to Whiteleaf, was keen to auspice the project in order to bring resources into the region. The regional service went through the formal process, on the town's behalf, to access funding.

Whiteleaf's population of around 6000 people is transient with 20 per cent of the population having moved to Whiteleaf in the past five years to gain employment in the mining and related industries. The demographics of the town reflect its industrial base. There is a predominance of younger families, with 30 per cent of the population fourteen years or under. The town is characterised by relative affluence, with a higher labour force participation rate and higher level of household income than is found in the Australian population generally. A small Australian Aboriginal population resides in a location about twenty kilometres from Whiteleaf. An older town (Old Town), with a small population and a very different demographic make-up, is approximately fifty kilometres away.

The social issues that Whiteleaf experiences are typical of towns where there is a transient population with young families living in a new environment separated from support systems. The shiftwork associated with the mine means that regular participation in the Whiteleaf Progress Association, the Hospital Board, and sporting activities is difficult. While the mining company provides infrastructure, including a sports ground, swimming pool, and an entertainment space, the facilities are not used by Aboriginal people, and young adults constantly complain of 'nothing to do'.

People living in Whiteleaf are aware of the misuse of recreational drugs and alcohol, but most would not regard it as a problem, more as entertainment on days off from working in the mine and a way of life in this isolated location. Although everyone agrees that Whiteleaf can be defined as a community, most residents don't regard Whiteleaf as their home. They refer to 'home' being in the location they came from and where their family and friends are. They regard their residence in Whiteleaf as short term, and they will move away if and when other employment opportunities arise.

Principle 1: Understanding communities

The first principle underpinning effective work with communities is to be able to understand and define the community that is to be the focus of the work. The two processes of defining and understanding are interrelated, but they are different. Understanding a community involves gaining knowledge about how the community functions, what organisations the community has, and how groups work together. Defining the community for the purpose of working on a particular task involves negotiating the geographic area and the particular group of people that will be involved in planning or developing the service or program.

Usually in community health and social care policy, the 'community' that is to be involved is ill-defined. It may refer to a group of people who live in a geographic area or consumers of a health or community service. Occasionally, there is no 'community' concept intended at all, and the term may be added because of the positive connotations of the word. Therefore, which 'community' we are working with is usually not apparent (Taylor et al. 2006a). This makes effective work in developing the communities' health and wellbeing all the more difficult.

Understanding the Whiteleaf community

The first issue then for the community worker is to identify the community he or she working with, which groups are involved, and who is to benefit from the initiative. In the Whiteleaf case example, there may be different ways to define who makes up the community. From the worker's perspective, the funding objectives state clearly that disadvantaged groups and all sectors within the community should be involved. Therefore it is likely that, for the purposes of this initiative, the worker will define the residents of Whiteleaf, along with the small groups of Aboriginal people who reside near Whiteleaf and the residents of Older Town nearby, as 'the community'. But is this how the Whiteleaf community understands and defines itself? Do residents in Whiteleaf include Aboriginal people in their understanding of their community?

In order to answer these questions, the community worker talks to people who know Whiteleaf, and develops an understanding of its structure and organisation, and of how people come together. The community worker listens to people, and learns about the divisions between those who work in the mine and those who don't. The separations between Whiteleaf's residents, the Australian Aboriginal population, and Old Town residents also become apparent. Residents themselves acknowledge the difficulty in getting disparate groups of people working together, and this has become a real difficulty when trying to develop the community. Listening to residents will assist the community worker in identifying the barriers to inclusive planning processes, but more importantly it will also highlight where there may be opportunities to overcome these barriers.

Issues in defining and understanding what 'community' is

The issues that the community worker will face in understanding and defining the community are in part due to the current usage of the term 'community' in health and human service policy. Historically, the term is used loosely and ambiguously in policy documents (Zakus and Lysack 1998, p. 2). It may be used to refer to a geographic location, a group of people with a particular health issue, an administrative region, or, in the case of general practice, a group of patients (Brown 1994, p. 338).

Communities are frequently arbitrarily defined by health and human service professionals, for pragmatic reasons, to suit the purposes of the task at hand, and there is usually a fundamental difference between the construction of community by members and non-members (Jewkes and Murcott 1996, p. 561). For example, restructuring administrative areas may bring together regions that have divergent interest groups and geographic areas that have few existing relationships, networks, or organisational links. Those people who reside in the areas may not regard the new region in any sense as a 'community'. This may not deter planners, who expect residents in these areas to work together as a 'community' to identify needs and priorities.

Frequently the term 'community' is used when there is no identifiable community being referred to at all, as the term has been comprehensively incorporated into mainstream language and its meaning has become obscured. Often we hear about the 'Australian community' as a way of talking about the total population of Australia (Bourke 2001a, p. 118).

There is another complication. The term 'community' has become aligned with a Utopian imagined perfect state of relationships offering warmth and security (Brent 2004, p. 213). Therefore, any kind of work with communities can be understood as a 'good thing' and to bring about an imagined state where people relate positively with each other.

CASE EXAMPLE 1.4

How to get a new consultative structure happening

Several towns in a region were to join together to establish a new consultative structure to replace each town's existing health and human services planning mechanisms. Service administrators were keen to create more efficiency in service delivery and more effective community participation. The towns are not only separated geographically, but they have very different industries and social structures. Because of this, they rarely connect for business or social reasons, and there has been ongoing rivalry between the local governments in each of the towns.

Think about it

➤ Why might administrators want to create a regional consultative structure?

➤ How might the towns involved view the move to disband the existing mechanisms and create new ones?

➤ What type of community participation in the consultative structures might service administrators have in mind?

➤ What types of community participation might the towns want?

We argue that this perception of 'community' as a good thing is a real problem when the process of working with communities inevitably involves tension over competing agendas and uncertainty about the outcomes of our work. So much so, that practitioners who become aware of community power struggles, exclusion of groups of people, and leadership battles may feel uncertain of their role and consider they are doing something wrong if they cannot solve these problems. Case example 1.4 illustrates tensions over competing agendas that are inevitable in community work.

Principle 2: Establishing relationships and partnerships

A common thread running through the research and theory about preventative health and social care initiatives is the need to work together. The importance of establishing relationships between communities, governments, and professionals in order to achieve health and social benefits for communities is continually highlighted. In fact, it is widely accepted that if residents of a community such as Whiteleaf were to become involved in identifying health or social issues, for example alcohol misuse, and were to work together with relevant professionals and governments to address the issue, then this would facilitate both health and social benefits for participants, and the community as a whole (WHO 2000). The World Health Organisation promotes the view that health and social wellbeing has become everybody's business (Steenbergen and El Ansari 2003).

The terms 'collaboration', 'partnerships', 'multi-disciplinary practice', and 'co-alitions' are used interchangeably in health and human service initiatives. The common element involved when using these terms is that informal and formal alliances are established and maintained between organisations, individuals, and communities for the purpose of achieving a common goal (Steenbergen and El Ansari 2003).

The argument for the establishment of partnerships rests on two foundations. First, the social and health issues facing providers, governments, and communities are now so serious that it is acknowledged that no one agency or organisation can solve, or even understand, problems alone. Planning and developing services and programs in the current environment is a highly complex activity, requiring a blend of technical expertise, knowledge, and skills from community members, local organisations, funding agencies, and professionals (Cheers 1998, p. 154). Second, forming partnerships and working relationships enables the workload and responsibility for the initiative to be shared, contributing to a greater likelihood of ownership of it from those who contribute. This, in turn, makes it likely that the initiative may be sustainable once the start-up period is complete (Shediac-Rizkallah and Bone 1998, p. 87).

Research suggests that successful partnerships involve clarity regarding the purpose of the relationship, and that the quality of the relationship is important. Factors such as whether or not there are mutual benefits, respect, honesty, sound communication, and sensitivity have an impact on whether or not partnerships persist. It has been found, for instance, that there is a need for greater emphasis on building trusting relationships across organisations and individuals within a context of unequal power relationships (Poland et al. 2005, p. 125). These researchers also note the importance of contextual factors on the progress of partnerships, including resource issues and differences between partners' organisational culture.

The belief by partners in the concept of 'collective efficacy' needs to be present if responsibility is to be shared. That is, members of the partnership need to

CASE EXAMPLE 1.5

Addressing youth homelessness

Agencies in a central city area began to meet regularly, facilitated by the local council, to coordinate their efforts in addressing youth homelessness. Those involved in working with the council included an organisation that distributed emergency financial relief, a youth group, a shelter for young adults, police representatives, and a large church organisation that provided a range of social care services. Meetings were held regularly and in the first year each of the people who attended achieved a better understanding of each of the agencies' roles and the problems young people faced. However, there was a high staff turnover and agency members had serious issues to address in their own agencies. Each of the groups had its own strategic plan, objectives, and tight timeframes. Attendance at meetings began to drop off as those people who had been involved in the early development of the group moved on. Eventually, while meetings continued to be regularly scheduled, there was only intermittent attendance, and a lack of clarity as to why the group had been convened.

Think about it

➤ What do you think might have been some of the potential benefits of having this group meet?
➤ Do you think any of these benefits were achieved?
➤ Do you think that the group should continue to meet?
➤ If it did, what might be its objectives?

believe that the combined efforts of the group are not only necessary for group members to obtain the desired shared goal, but also that all members are capable of doing and willing to do their share of the work (Johnson et al. 2003, p. 70). There must also be a continual focus on achieving the outputs required from the partnership. Too often the reasons for forming the partnership and the benefits it was to provide become lost along the way.

Case example 1.5 illustrates the last point. Sometimes meetings between partners become routine rather than focused on achieving outcomes.

Establishing partnerships in Whiteleaf

In the Whiteleaf case example 1.3, the process of understanding Whiteleaf goes hand in hand with the formation of partnerships and working relationships. The worker finds that there is difficulty in getting people to come together to plan for the new initiative because of the separations in the community. These separations are among older and newer residents, those who work for the mine and those who don't, and Whiteleaf residents and the Aboriginal people. The worker needs to accept these divisions and make contact with people in the different groups, and ask for advice about how to overcome these divisions. This will involve working through the key people as well as including those who may have been overlooked in the past.

Whiteleaf has been targeted to receive funding on the basis of the relatively low level of existing health infrastructure and its difficulty in attracting a health and human service workforce, rather than because of an awareness of health issues and the capacity and capability for the community to address the issues. Possibly most residents in Whiteleaf are not aware of the likelihood of serious health conditions arising in the future because of aspects of their lifestyles. If they are aware of these, they might find it difficult to address them because of time, resources, or a lack of knowledge. Alternatively, residents might be well aware of the health and social issues, but regard the solution as more services, including social workers, community nurses, and doctors.

It is likely that the majority of residents will hold very different perspectives on health and human services issues from those of the community worker. Sharing knowledge, skills, and resources will be essential, but first residents will need to want to be involved. Clearly, involving residents in the processes of identifying what the issues are is fundamental if the residents are to see the initiative as useful and belonging to the community.

A common incentive for Whiteleaf residents to become involved is that all groups are very keen on receiving funding in order to develop new projects. When asked whether or not Whiteleaf would like to be involved in the bid for funding, the Whiteleaf Progress Association members thought that developing appropriate programs for young adults was a high priority. After school and on weekends, young people were without adult support while their parents worked. It was very difficult to organise shiftwork so that adults were available to provide supervision, and young people were thought to be at risk of drug and alcohol misuse.

In spite of the desire to access funding and put in place some new programs and services, the residents are pessimistic. Several years ago, Whiteleaf tried unsuccessfully to get ongoing funding for the family counselling outreach worker. In spite of people's efforts, the service was discontinued and residents came away thinking that they didn't have the skills and knowledge required to put forward their case and adequately demonstrate the need for the service. Consequently, the worker is now faced with genuine concern from community members that getting involved in more planning may result in a lot of hard work with uncertain outcomes.

These are some of the issues in developing relationships in Whiteleaf. The worker will listen to these concerns and explore with the residents the types of programs that may be established, their relative value to the community, how sustainable they might be, and how much work for residents will be involved. Then the worker will need to negotiate within their organisation and with the funding body to ensure that Whiteleaf's priorities can be accommodated.

Issues in establishing and maintaining partnerships

Those who are engaged in developing services will bring different perspectives, experiences, backgrounds, technical expertise, attitudes, and values to their work. This blending of people's knowledge and skills is in Australian Aboriginal ways of knowing likened to the process of bringing the fresh and salty water together (Juanita Sherwood, personal communication, 17 July 2004). Different elements come together in a way that creates a new substance and a shared understanding. This shared understanding then provides the common ground or context in which development can occur, and is a precursor to partners being able to work effectively together. The challenge in working together is to blend the knowledge and experience of those involved to bring about effective, relevant, and long-lasting programs and services.

However, like all processes that involve working with people, there are complexities in establishing and maintaining working relationships. Essentially partnerships depend on people remaining committed to them. They require the energy, enthusiasm, and commitment of one or more 'champions' (Poland et al. 2005, p. 125). While formal written partnership statements between organisations that are displayed in office entrances are in vogue, they only demonstrate organisational commitment to partnerships, but do not bring them about. It is the nature of the relationships between people, particularly in relation to power-sharing and communication, that is all important (Rifkin et al. 2000, pp. x–xi).

In writing about health development, often a concept of partnership is employed that equates with people's willing involvement in projects that are bereft of intense power struggles, shifting alliances, and disagreements about goals and objectives. While we know anecdotally that this is not the case, studies that analyse partnership processes with respect to the negotiation of power struggles are few and far between. Case studies of rural development illustrate that respecting people's abilities may be fundamental to effective partnerships.

[C]ase studies of effective rural development speak for themselves, eloquently, movingly and persuasively. They show us that approaches to rural development that respect the inherent capabilities, intelligence and responsibility of rural people and that systematically build on their experience have a reasonable chance of making significant advances in improving those people's lives. (Krishna et al. 1997, p. 2)

Practice tip 1.1

The Participate in Health website www.participateinhealth.org.au has relevant information to promote community participation.

It is very important to remember that in working with well-established communities of place or of interest, there is a context, a background, and a way of doing things that have persisted over long periods of time. There is a collective world view including values and attitudes, and stories the community tells about itself. Trying to work to implement a program or a new service will need to be considered against this backdrop.

Understanding different types of communities involves accepting the patterns of interaction and the collective world view of the community where it exists. There must be a willingness to work with these realities and not against them. We do this by establishing sound working relationships that involve respecting the knowledge and skills of each partner.

In a newer community, for example, a new housing estate on the fringes of a large city, it is almost the reverse situation. There may be few established ways of relating, no background of shared activity, few organisational structures, and only the beginnings of a collective world view. In this case, it is working with the community to help develop structures, networks, and collective views.

SUMMARY

The case example of Whiteleaf demonstrates the two fundamental principles that underpin community work. If Whiteleaf residents and those living in the surrounding area are to make effective use of the funding opportunity and get relevant programs up and running, there will need to be effective partnerships between people. Those who have the knowledge about preventative health programs and how to implement them have a crucial role to play. So, too, do the people who live and work in Whiteleaf, who understand the town, its leaders, social organisation, and those who are excluded and included in social life. It is the partnerships that lead to the community understanding the health development opportunity and the community worker understanding how the community ticks.

This book is all about these issues. It is about how and why communities of place and of interest get involved in developing and maintaining health and human services and programs and the types of working relationships that are needed if the programs are to be effective.

USEFUL WEBSITES

The Sustainable Communities Network provides an introduction to sustainable
community action: http://www.sustainable.org/

The Community Development Society is an international organisation promoting
sound practice and research in community development: http://comm-dev.
org/

Community Development Australia is an organisation to promote community
development: http://www.cds.org.au/

The International community development association is a non-government
organisation committed to building a global network of people and
organisations working toward social justice through community
development: http://www.health.state.mn.us/divs/hpcd/chp/hpkit/index.
htm#whyapp

The Aspen Institute round table on community change: http://www.aspeninstitute.
org/site/c.huLWJeMRKpH/b.612045/k.4BA8/Roundtable_on_Community_
Change.htm

The Participate in Health website, maintained by the Victorian Government,
has publications on community participation in health: http://www.
participateinhealth.org.au/

CHAPTER 2

What is Community?

Introduction

Our starting point in community health and social care development is to ask an empirical question—what is the community I am working with and what are its qualities that will impact upon the programs or services that I am trying to develop? This and the next two chapters, Aboriginal understandings of community, and understanding community capacity, provide the tools to answer these questions.

In this book, it is communities rather than individuals or organisations that are the centre of attention. Working with the interactions, networks, structures, and processes that make up the community requires different practice skills and frameworks than working with individuals.

Much of the research about community and community functioning used in this chapter has been undertaken in rural communities, because the patterns of interaction can be seen clearly in these settings. However, the concepts are illustrated through giving examples relevant to community health and social care development in rural, regional, and urban communities, and of communities of interest.

First, we discuss different ways that community has been understood, as a community of place, a common interest community, and as a social system. Then we present an evidence-based definition that has been developed for public health practice. Five elements of community structure and functioning are examined in the second section of the chapter:

➤ the local society;
➤ the community field;
➤ community structures and power networks;
➤ horizontal and vertical links;
➤ strong and weak ties; and
➤ community narratives.

Defining community

The concept of community is deeply rooted in the history of sociological thought, and in this thinking there are two generally recognised ways that community is understood. These are the geographic or locality-based understanding and the relational concept of community. These components, geography and relationships, are present to a greater or lesser degree in most theoretical understandings of community, and Heller's definition reflects this.

> Community as a locality refers to the territorial or geographic notion of community—the neighbourhood, town or city. The second meaning of community, the relational community, refers to qualities of human interaction and social ties that draw people together (Heller 1989, p. 3).

The following section examines each of these understandings in more detail and defines a community of place, a community of interest, and a community as a social system.

Community as locality and interactions

Sociological definitions of community have usually emphasised a given territory or a commonly shared geographical area. Hillery (1955) conducted a content analysis of ninety-four definitions of community in the sociological literature and found that sixty-nine agreed that social interaction, area, and a common tie or ties were fundamental to community life. He then attempted theoretical development of this apparent consensus about a definition of community by comparing community types (which he calls 'communal organisations') such as cities, villages, and institutions (Hillery 1968).

Sociologists usually agree that community exists in small rural towns because interactions can and do occur between people acting together meeting their common interests. However, there is less agreement about whether community exists in cities and other places where people have access to a range of relationships and multiple interactions outside the locality. In cities, for example, people may be geographically separated from their place of employment and perhaps from their preferred shopping, and their family and friends (Scherer 1972, p. 19). This is true now for some rural dwellers as well, because people travel to regional centres for employment and for business (Bourke 2001a). So where there are multiple interactions away from where people live, can community still exist?

Wilkinson (1991) argues strongly in the affirmative. His argument, based in social interaction theory (Kaufman 1959), is that essentially community comes about because of natural processes of social interaction in a location. Wilkinson's view is that where there are ongoing interactions between people in a given locality, and where there are locally oriented networks, organisations, and structures that support these interactions, then community can exist. Both location and interactions are fundamental to the interactional perspective of community.

Community may exist in a neighbourhood in a city, a regional centre, a rural town, or a tropical island tourist resort where there is a commonly identified place in which people interact with others. Proximity is one factor in building community; as people talk to their next-door neighbour, they may pass each other going to the local shop, or share information about the locality. In areas where people do not live close to each other, they may regularly visit a location for shopping or health facilities, and patterned interactions occur. So, although the nature of the territory is an important component, it is interactions that are the substance of community and the place to start looking for it. Community can exist where there are patterned interactions between people acting together in the common concerns of life.

Activity 2.1

Defining community

Think of a neighbourhood, a town or a group of people that you would define as a community. What are the important elements that make up this community?

Practice tip 2.1

Remember that defining and understanding a community are two different things. A community may be defined as such for administrative purposes, but may not show the important elements of a community.

Community of place

The term 'community of place' is used in writing about rural communities in the sociological literature to describe a community that is bounded geographically and includes social interactions among people who live in the area. Drawing on Wilkinson's work about community interaction, Cheers and Luloff (2001, p. 130) define communities of place as 'characterised by three components: locality, local society, and a process of locality-oriented collective actions characteristically called the 'community field'.

According to Wilkinson (1991, pp. 2–3) there are three elements involved in defining a community of place. The first is a locality, and this is a geographical area or territory where people live and meet their daily needs together. In order for a geographical area to become a locality, it needs to be demarcated by more or less locally agreed boundaries. The boundaries are usually dynamic and may be constructed differently, depending, to a degree, on the purposes of construction, and the movement of relationships. For example, a community may be defined as the major town and all the smaller towns for health service provision, but for all other purposes, the smaller towns may not been seen as making up the community.

Within the defined boundaries, there is a local society, which is all the structures, organisations, and networks enabling residents to meet their business and social needs, and providing access to services. The third element is the locally oriented social interactions that are the essence of community. These are the relationships between people that occur naturally as people come together to meet their needs. It is not the intensity of the interactions or whether they are satisfying from an emotional point of view that is important. What is important to definitions of community is that they exist and are patterned.

Activity 2.2

A community of place: Whiteleaf

The case example about Whiteleaf in Chapter 1 (1.3) illustrates a community of place. All the residents of Whiteleaf agree that Whiteleaf is the place where they have friendships, regular contact with networks and organisations, and service agencies. There are regular interactions with health professionals, shop keepers, and local council staff. People who live in Whiteleaf join sporting clubs, some belong to church groups, and may socialise at the hotel or the club. Informally, they meet each other at the shops and when they pick up children from school.

Think about it

➤ Are there patterned interactions between Whiteleaf residents?
➤ Is there a local society in Whiteleaf?
➤ What common interests might Whiteleaf residents have?

Community as a common interest group

Adopting Guterbock's (1999, p. 92) definition, communities can also be viewed as groups of people who share a consistent set of interactions around a common interest, whether it be an economic, social, political, spiritual or cultural interest. Communities of interest may come together for a specific time-limited purpose, such as advocating for a new service or lobbying a political party around an issue prior to an election. An example is an environmental group who lobby against a proposed freeway through the neighbourhood.

On the other hand, some communities of interest are enduring, and these are likely to be those that engage people around aspects of their lives that are important, such as their faith, sexual identity, or culture. For example, people with similar cultural and ethnic backgrounds frequently interact as a community

CASE EXAMPLE 2.1

Community of interest: Bfriend

Bfriend is a program of UnitingCare Wesley Adelaide that is in its eleventh year. The heart of the work of Bfriend is to support men and women, of all ages, who are questioning their sexuality or gender identity. That is done primarily through linking them up with trained volunteers who are same sex attracted or transgender people themselves. We try to offer a safe space for people to make more sense of who they are and what their new thoughts are about their identity and sexuality that they've kept buried for a long time.

People talk about the gay, lesbian, bisexual, and transgender (GLBT) community or the queer community as if it's a single entity and it's not. How I think of it is many communities and individuals within a broader thing that's called the GLBT community.

For me, what characterises my community is a sense of belonging and connection and having hope for the future that, by finding a place to belong, actually allows us to be acknowledged for who we really are, to be with people who don't question who we are. It gives us a chance to make friends, build relationships, and be surrounded by love and support and this makes the world a much safer place to be. So then, when we step outside of those safe environments and we're affected by other people's suspicion and fear then we've got a safe place to come back to for respite.

But within that notion of community there are differences. For some people it's not always safe. I think particularly of people who identify as bisexual or transgender are often treated with suspicion in the GLBT community. So for me, the notion of community as a safe place and a place to find belonging is my ideal about community. But within that, we're faced with all the challenges that any community is faced with about accepting and being alongside people who either look different to us or who act differently or who have different values or whatever, so there's always that incredible tension.

Bfriend runs monthly opportunities for people to meet other people in a safe social place. The community is made up of folk who have as many and diverse interests as any community in Australia. We find ways to engage in those passions like anybody else, so you'll get groups around bush walking, photography, dancing, discussion groups, and a whole plethora of things that have us being engaged. I think at the heart of that is friendship, so that the friendships that we form will sustain us in our lives. Community is built by being friends to each other and that gives a sense of meaning.

Think about it

➤ Are there patterned interactions between people in this community of interest?
➤ What are the common interests on which this community is built?
➤ Is there a local society?
➤ Is there a geographic territory in which the community exists?

providing for the social, cultural, and spiritual needs of their members. An example of a community that provides for a wide range of their member's needs is the Aboriginal 'culture community' in Australia. Culture community will be explored in depth in the next chapter.

Communities of interest may be bounded geographically, but they may not be, and people may belong to more than one community. Generally, communities of interest and communities of place coexist in multiple layers. For example, in an urban neighbourhood that is a community of place, there may be people who belong to the neighbourhood as well as a culture or faith community.

Communities of interest will always exhibit two elements of a community of place. They will have social interactions enabling people to act together around their common interests and concerns, express their identity, and friendships. There will also be a local society, with networks, patterns of relationships, organisations, and other structures that support these interactions.

A debatable point in defining a community of interest is whether or not interactions must be face to face. Some people would argue that groups of people who share conversations and form relationships by email and the Internet, but who never meet, can be called 'cyber-communities'. What do you think?

The example of a community of interest (Case example 2.1) is provided by Truffy Maginnis at Bfriend, a program of UnitingCare Wesley Adelaide.

Community as a social system

In some of the health-promotion literature, community is defined as a social system drawing on the application of social systems theory (Parsons 1951) to community analysis by Warren (1978). Social systems theory is useful in health promotion in order to understand the patterns of interactions that are built up over time in health systems and communities. Understanding these links between elements of health systems, and communities' organisations is central in assessing community needs, resources, and readiness for introduction of health-promotion programs (Rissel and Bracht 1999; Walter 2005).

A fundamental principle underpinning social systems theory is that there is order in the interrelationships of the various components of the system over time.

> A social system is a structural organisation of the interaction of units that endures through time. It has both internal and external aspects relating the system to its environment and its units to each other. It can be distinguished from the surrounding environment, performing a function called boundary maintenance. It tends to maintain an equilibrium in the sense that it adapts to changes from outside the system in such a way as to minimise the impact of the change on the organisational structure and to regularise the subsequent relationships. (Warren 1978, p. 136)

Warren (1978) applies this principle of structural organisation to analyse community functioning. He says that over time, a community's social interactions follow systemic patterns and these become structures or units of interaction. A community contains a number of these units that can be understood as subsystems. In this sense, a community becomes a 'system of systems'. The analysis of the interrelation of subsystems within the community and the relationship between local subsystems and those that extend beyond the community is an examination of patterns of ordered interaction. These patterns of interaction within the community are called horizontal patterns, and those patterns that extend beyond the community are called vertical patterns. Here is an example of a community health social system.

CASE EXAMPLE 2.2

A community health social system

The community health centre is well linked both within the local community and in the broader health system. The centre is located in a busy shopping complex, and is a stopping-off point for people to gain information and renew their relationships with other community members. Staff members have positions on the local government health planning groups, and have regular contacts with the schools in the area. Within the broader health system, the community health centre is represented on the regional planning group, and the coordinator attends bimonthly state level community health planning meetings.

Think about it

➤ What are some of the elements of the community health centre social system?
➤ What are the some of the patterned interactions?
➤ Where are the horizontal and vertical links?

In traditional social systems theory (Parsons 1951), the term 'boundary maintenance' refers to the way in which the system maintains consistent patterns with those elements that are within the system. A clear boundary is maintained between those components that are within the system and those that are not. A community health centre may have links with health-related organisations, but not with the tourism service sector. This helps to keep the elements of the system together and focused around the interactions that are important—in this case building community health.

Another term used in systems theory is that of 'equilibrium', and this refers to the inherent tendency that systems have to maintain a balance between elements within the system. Again, this helps to keep the system functioning. However, Warren (1978) considers that there are some problems with applying both the concepts of equilibrium and boundary maintenance to communities. Community subsystems are based on social interactions between people, and how these interactions can be integrated in such a way as to maintain a system's equilibrium is difficult to understand. Wilkinson (1998) considered that the concept of a community having a self-regulatory system and an inherent maintenance tendency was particularly problematic. Social interactions between people are fluid, dynamic, often unpredictable, and may be strongly affected by chance factors, and may not, in the sense used in social systems theory, be self-regulating.

Walter (2005 p. 68) expands the social systems concept to include potentially all the relationships between organisations and people at every level in the community.

> I refer to community as multidimensional to describe the way in which the various dimensions that characterize community—such as people and organisations, consciousness, actions, and context are integrally related with one another, forming the whole that is community. To develop an understanding of community, then, we need to articulate, visualize, and examine the unique qualities exhibited by each of these dimensions and how these dimensions come together to make up the complex and dynamic system of community.

This concept of a multidimensional system is useful for people who work with communities because it acknowledges the multiple stakeholders with diverse interests and complex power relationships within communities. These power relationships result in some voices being dominant and others being marginalised. This orientation ensures that professionals enlarge what is taken into account in orienting practice, and reveals additional avenues for practice activity.

An evidence-based definition of community

In all three of these understandings of community, social interactions and relationships between people are fundamental. Research conducted in the United States, asking people how they understood 'community', also confirmed that social interaction was the principal element of the definition (MacQueen et al. 2001, p. 1929).

CASE EXAMPLE 2.3

An evidence-based definition of community for public health practice

Source MacQueen et al. 2001, p. 1929

Residents from diverse socio-economic groups in different cities and states of America were asked how they defined community. The analysis found five elements were central, each of which involved some aspect of face-to-face interaction. The elements were: a commonly agreed upon place; sharing common interests; joint action; relationships between people; and social complexity. Community was defined as 'a group of people with diverse characteristics who are linked by social ties, share common perspectives, and engage in joint action in geographical locations or settings'.

Think about it

➤ Which do you think are the most important elements of this definition of community?

➤ What elements do you think are essential for community to exist?

A normative view of community

Brent (2004), Bourke (2001b), Edwards et al. (2003), and Walter (2005, p. 68) all note that there is a tendency in some health and social development policy to view community only as a 'positive', and strive for the development of these positive characteristics. The normative view sees community as a structure within which people have a sense of solidarity—being in things together—and this creates a sense of belonging to each other. This in turn results in positive affirmations for people because of their membership of the community.

Cleaver (2001, p. 44) is particularly critical of this 'solidarity' model of community, on which, he says, much economic and social development intervention in developing countries is based. His view is that the model leads to the assumption

CASE EXAMPLE 2.4

A community health project in South Africa

Source: Kelly and Vlaenderen 1996, p. 1236

A collaborative project, aimed to develop centres to train community health personnel, had been funded by an international donor. On presentation of the proposal, the donor considered the participation of the community in the process of drafting the proposal was inadequate. However, 'until fairly recently, *[people had been]* deeply committed to political struggle rather than co-operation. The history of this struggle and the legacy of the past, inevitably continue to create a degree of suspicion and mistrust and will arguably do so for some time to come'.

that there is always some commonality of interest between people, in spite of social stratification, economic inequalities, and diverse interests. This view simplifies the complexities of community development and leads to the 'myth of community', in which community is seen as a state of positive and peaceful social relationships.

Brent (2004, p. 213) suggests that a more 'complex analysis is needed to unravel the unsubstantial but nonetheless powerful characteristics of community'. Communities are neither always a source of peace and prosperity for their members, neither are they the source of all the problems that people experience (Kretzmann 2000). There are elements of community structure and functioning that assist in developing community health and wellbeing, and there are some elements that may work against this. It is important for communities and those who work with them to understand these factors.

The development of a community-based health service in South Africa shows how important it is to acknowledge how the real conflicts between community groups and political struggles will make cooperative action to address issues very difficult (Kelly and Vlaenderen 1996, p. 1236).

Practice tip 2.2

Usually it is unhelpful to identify a community as 'functional' or 'dysfunctional'. It is much more complex than that—consider the following view of a research participant.

We are lucky that we have a very close community and because we cover so many towns, everyone seems to work in together. In times of trouble and tragedy, community is a total commitment and you have to go through that to appreciate what is out there. Communities are so strong and that can be overpowering as well; if you step out of line that can be devastating in a small town. (Community member)

Elements of structure and functioning of communities

This book uses community interaction theory as the primary theoretical approach to underpin community health and social care development. Wilkinson (1970, 1972, 1991), with his focus on community interaction, set the foundation for the body of knowledge that we refer to as community interaction theory. Bridger and Luloff (1999), Cheers and Luloff (2001), Sharp (2001), and Carroll et al. (2006) have all contributed to its development. This theoretical approach has been chosen because it provides us with concepts to help us understand the community structures and processes that are an essential part of building effective interactions, networks, and relationships. It is the strengthening of relationships to allow communities to take action in community and social care development that is all-important.

A community comes together, across sectors through purposive locality-oriented collective actions. The essence of community is social interaction. People who live together in the same geographic area may think of themselves as a community, but they do not necessarily constitute a community unless they act together (Wilkinson 1991, p. 3). Therefore, in order to understand a community, whether it is a community of place, a community of interest, or a community system, we need to understand how the community comes together and acts. To do this, we must consider:

➤ the local society;
➤ the community field;
➤ community structures (including power networks);
➤ horizontal and vertical patterns of interaction;
➤ strong and weak ties; and
➤ community narratives.

All these elements are apparent in communities of place, whether they are small rural or remote communities, inner city neighbourhoods, or new developments in outer metropolitan areas. The same elements are also evident in communities of interest.

A local society

In a community of place, a local society enables residents to meet their social, material, economic, and business needs, and provides access to services. 'A local society is a comprehensive network of associations for meeting common needs and expressing common interests' (Wilkinson 1991, p. 2). For example, in the example of Whiteleaf (Case example 1.3), there are sporting and social clubs, and businesses that facilitate interactions around a common purpose. This is the same in a community of interest. The Bfriend organisation (Case example 2.1) has writing groups where people meet around their common interests.

There are many ways that social structures and networks can be organised and can connect people, but it is the existence of these that enable interaction. In Whiteleaf, the important local structures bringing people together to plan community development and health service delivery are the Hospital Board and the Whiteleaf Progress Association. There are also informal networks developed at work and through participation in sporting events.

A local society is marked by several more or less distinctive social fields where locality-oriented interactions are directed towards achieving specific goals for residents. A social field is dynamic and constantly changing as the needs of the community change (Wilkinson 1991, p. 36).

The key elements of a local society are:

➤ the local actors or participants;
➤ the groups, networks, and associations through which the action occurs; and
➤ the distinctive social fields within the local society.

In Whiteleaf, for example, there is a health social field. This involves people from the hospital, the mining company, and volunteer groups working together to achieve a specific objective—improvement in health care.

The community field

One of the most powerful concepts from the community interactional theorists is that of the community field. Wilkinson (1970, 1991) develops the concept of the community field as an unbounded whole, with a constantly changing structure that is used to bring people together to solve development problems of the entire community. It is the presence of the community field that makes a local society in a geographic place a community.

CASE EXAMPLE 2.5

The Greenbee community links

Even though there were many changes, there were still people who had lived in the inner city suburb Greenbee for generations, and they valued their strong links with the locale. Over the years, a number of organisations had developed where people could join together around local issues. The family history association ran regular events where the newer residents could meet the long-term residents. The development group had put 'story boards' at various places in the city, which told of the significance of the area to the traditional Aboriginal owners. The school, with the help of volunteers, had recorded the names of all the teachers who had taught there since its establishment.

There had been many changes in the style of housing over the years, with the single bungalow making way for apartment blocks. There were now younger families moving into the area, renovating the older houses, and buying the apartments. Residents had worked together to lobby for improved housing development planning processes, and had successfully lobbied for purpose-built accommodation for older people so that they could stay in the area. The local council was supportive of including both the long-term and newer residents in planning for the community.

Think about it

➤ How do you think the community field evolves in Greenbee?
➤ What are the issues that need to be overcome in bringing people together to plan?
➤ What structures facilitate people coming together?

Wilkinson argues that the development of particular social fields in a community, such as the health or education social fields, does not necessarily lead to the development of a community field, because it is the actions for the common good across the special interest fields that define the community field. The community field is the linking and coordinating of activities that occur within social fields bringing information, experience, resources, and energy together to solve community issues or plan development.

'The short answer to why the community "hangs together" is that a community field tends to occur where people live together and interact on matters concerning their common interest in the locality' (Wilkinson 1991, p. 37). The basic characteristic of the community field, then, is the purposive interaction across diverse social fields that facilitates awareness of local concerns and enhances the flow of information and financial resources.

Community structures and power networks

Community interaction theory identifies different types of structures and power networks that operate in communities. These 'ideal types' are not likely to exist in the real world in their pure form. It is more likely that structures will overlap, and there may be elements of more than one type of structure.

Identifying the types of structures and power networks that operate in communities is useful because it tells us about who has the power to make decisions, whether or not there are likely to be competing interest groups, and whether it will be possible for the community to work together across sectors. Drawing on community interaction theorists (Kaufman 1959; Wilkinson 1970,

1972, 1991, 1998), Sharp (2001, p. 403) shows ways in which community power structures will affect the capacity the community has to bring social fields together and create a community field. If, for example, there are enduring power struggles over resources between the health and education sectors in a community, then it is going to be difficult for groups to come together and consider the interests of the community as a whole. Community health or social care development involving cross-sector activities will require considerable facilitation.

Community structures

Wilkinson (1998) presents four types of community structures: the integrated; the segmented; the factionalised; and the amorphous community. The integrated type has well-linked and coordinated community activities across all of the social fields or interest sectors. The segmented community structure has well-linked and coordinated social fields, but very few links with other sectors. For example, the health and human services social field in a community may be well-linked within the field, but have no links to other social fields, such as the tourism social field. In the factionalised community structure, there are divisions among groups of people right across the community according to culture, socio-economic status, or political persuasion. For example, professionals may link with other professionals in other social fields rather than with other health or human services organisations. The amorphous community structure has little or no structure at all, and this type occurs in emerging or dissolving communities.

Community power structures

Sharp (2001) developed a typology of community power structures: the pyramid; factional; coalitional; and amorphous. The pyramidal structure concentrates power in a single cohesive group, and other groups are brought together through networks that link to this group. In the factional structure, social fields are connected to two (or more) networks. Each of these networks holds power to make decisions about the resources it controls, but there are few, if any, networks that can link the factions. In the coalitional structure, power is relatively decentralised and shared among groups who are working together in fluid coalitions. In a community with an amorphous power network structure, there may be hardly any power concentrations because there are few enduring coalitions between groups, organisations, or sectors. This may because there is a high turnover of population, or industrial expansion or decline.

Here is an example of the community structures and power networks that operate in Mountown.

CASE EXAMPLE 2.6

Mountown: a divided community?

Residents in Mountown, an island suburb of a large city, argue that it is a factionalised community with some people supporting the economic development of the island and some supporting the retention of the 'laid back lifestyle'. Over the years, these two groups have become consolidated, and special-interest groups have become aligned with one or other of the factions. While there are many organisations, such as the Surf Lifesaving Organisation, the Theatre Group, and the Wild Life Carers Group, membership of the groups tends to be dominated by those from one or other of the factions.

One of the residents explains how the community functions: 'I think what is interesting is that when there is a serious threat to the community with a flood or a fire, one of the things that becomes very evident is that the groups who would never be seen talking to each other are in fact there standing beside each other passing the sand bags or whatever, so in some ways you know there's exposed moments where one's sense of community becomes redefined again. Everybody knows that they can contribute. People are connected through systems like the State Emergency Service that is based on volunteers and there are neighbourhood captains, and in some way all organisations and people are connected in. There are times when the connections between people, organisations and interest groups become weaker, and perhaps that's because when things are flying along pretty well'.

Think about it

➤ What kind of community structure do you think Mountown has—integrated, segmented, factionalised, or amorphous?
➤ What kind of power network do you think that Mountown has—pyramidal, coalitional, factional, or amorphous?

Horizontal and vertical patterns of interaction

The concepts of vertical and horizontal patterning of systems interactions (Warren 1978) are useful to understand the potential for collaborative activity both within and external to the community. Horizontal patterning is the relationships of the community's various social units and subsystems, such as sporting groups, women's organisations, and service clubs, to each other. Vertical patterning is the connections between community's social units to extra-community systems, such as the relationship between local government and the state government (Martinez-Brawley 2000; Warren 1978, p. 243).

In a health or human services project, such as the establishment of a neighbourhood centre or a health-promotion project, there is a need for a balance of vertical and horizontal patterning of interaction. Vertical interactions between subsystems are necessary to maintain links with the outside world, bringing in information about the effectiveness of particular programs, how they might be adapted to suit the community, and financial resources to run the program. In health and social care development, professionals external to the community provide links to information about funding programs and skills necessary to develop and manage services.

The horizontal patterns of interactions are the ones that occur within the community, built up through relationships among friends, neighbours, and families. These interactions enable the community to function. They influence and are influenced by the community networks and the power structures, and are dynamic and complex. Here is an example of horizontal and vertical patterns of interaction.

CASE EXAMPLE 2.7

Horizontal and vertical patterns of interaction: Greentown

The neighbourhood centre in Greentown is an important part of the social infrastructure in the community. Greentown is a new suburb, on the fringes of a large city, and while it has some public facilities, sporting clubs, and shops, there are few locations where organisations can hold meetings and people can drop in to chat and get information about local events. The centre is run by a group of volunteers from different groups in the community, all of whom have an interest in developing the community. The centre has strong links with social service and other government departments based in the city, and regularly invites representatives to give updates about new initiatives. The centre is also part of a national network advocating for better resourcing for neighbourhood centres.

Think about it

➤ What are the horizontal links drawn upon by the neighbourhood centre?
➤ What are the vertical links?
➤ What factors might facilitate the development of horizontal and vertical links at the neighbourhood centre?

Strong and weak ties

The concept of strong and weak interpersonal ties, both within the community and external to it, is useful to understand more about how communities can become involved in community health and social care development. According to Granovetter (1973), the strength of a tie (or relationship) is a combination of the amount of time, the emotional intensity, the intimacy, and the reciprocal services that characterise the tie. For example, a community may be strongly aligned around family and close relationships, and this may result in its being partitioned into cliques, with every person tied to every other person in his or her clique, and to none outside it. These ties become binding in the sense that they build cohesion, and in the process separate groups and families from each other. Strong ties are most often found within a community.

Weak ties are those between people who have occasional contacts. The relationships are not emotionally intense and there is limited investment of time. In communities of place and communities of interest, people who are new to the

CASE EXAMPLE 2.8

Strong and weak ties: The Italian community

Community members in a regional city are proud of their Italian heritage, culture, and traditions. There are many strong relationships across family groupings and ties among people whose families came from the same regions in Italy. While community members are interested in maintaining their cultural traditions, they are also interested in advancing the community by providing relevant services. A project that the current management committee is pursuing is to provide accommodation for older adults. In order to do this, they have invited people onto the management committee who are not Italian, and have no strong ties to the community, but possess financial management skills and experience in designing accommodation facilities.

Think about it

➤ Where are the strong ties in this community?
➤ Where are the weak ties?
➤ Why is a balance of strong and weak ties important in developing this community?

community and those who spend a large amount of their time outside it may have mainly weak ties within the community, but strong ties outside of it (Granovetter 1973, p. 1361).

Health and social care development in communities of place, if it is to be successful, requires a balance of strong and weak ties (Cheers 1993, p. 66). Many small rural communities or communities of interest may have numerous strong ties that involve intimate and continuing relations among family members and friends within the community. In these communities, there may be few weak ties with people in the community or with experts outside it. It is possible that these communities become inward-looking and draw on their own resources. Weak ties are important because they can build new relationships, altering patterns of interaction and adding resources that may be needed for development. Case example 2.8 is of a community of interest and the strong and weak ties that assist development.

Practice tip 2.3

Often people who are new to a community have an important role to play in bringing in new ideas and perspectives. It may be important to ensure that these people can have a say, as they may open up debate.

Community narratives

Community narratives are the stories people in a community tell about their community to themselves and to others. The stories, reflecting the dominant community traditions, values and attitudes, help define the community for members and distinguish it from other communities.

Both in communities of interest and of place, there are narratives that support or work against participation in health and human services. Communities may have made significant financial contributions and given time, expertise, and provided governance for a whole range of community services, including hospitals, older persons' accommodation, health centres, neighbourhood centres and other services, such as men's sheds, to name just a few. In this case, people's contributions are consistent with communitywide narratives about how the community functions, and that service and community viability is dependent on their contribution (Taylor, Williams et al. 2006). On the other hand, there may be narratives that hinder community health and social care development.

The following comment by a research participant illustrates a tradition of service to the community that is embedded in family and community history.

I guess my motivation to contribute is about being local and being involved in everything. It is instilled in you to do things. My mother was very community minded and my grandmother also. It is a part of your way of life if your mother and father have modelled it. We get things done in this community by working together. (Hospital board member)

When events challenge or threaten community viability, community narratives often come to the fore. For example, a community had a strong tradition of civic participation and volunteering to support its health services, because the health care industry was a major employer in the town. When there was talk of closing the small local hospital, people from all sectors of the community worked together to keep it open.

CASE EXAMPLE 2.9

Community narratives: Browntown

Source: Cheers et al. 2004

In Browntown, the dominant narrative was of a lucky, stable community, which has been well enough endowed by location, physical resources, and climate to be reasonably economically secure. A secondary narrative was that continuity and stability are more important than change. A subversive narrative told of a small clique of powerful leaders holding the economic growth of the community back. A latent narrative was that if change and growth are in the interests of local businesses, who had latent power in their own right, they would support it, if necessary against the leadership clique. Finally, the emergent narrative in this community, led by a small subversive group of entrepreneurs, was that economic diversification (and, by implication, change and growth) should be pursued because it is in the interests of the community as a whole.

Think about it

➤ What influence do you think that dominant narrative has in this community?
➤ At what times do you think that the subversive narratives might be heard?
➤ Do you think it is likely that emergent narratives might take hold in this community?

We all work together to protect our hospital. I am interested in the future of what is happening with our hospital because I have always lived here and I rely on it so much. If we lose our hospital, it is amazing what happens to a town. A lot of towns have closed the hospitals down and people say that nothing will change; but it does. You lose a lot of other small businesses; eventually they just seem to move out. We've lost so much; if it wasn't for the hospital, the school and the town wouldn't be viable at all. (Hospital volunteer)

Community narratives evolve over time and are affected by changing community circumstances and leadership. Written histories of the community, annual reports of organisations, and community promotional material usually identifies some community narratives. Research in rural South Australia identified five kinds of narratives (Cheers et al. 2004):

➤ Dominant narratives are the strongest stories in that they have most influence over how people construct the community.
➤ Secondary narratives have less influence and are consistent with the dominant ones.
➤ Subversive narratives challenge the dominant ones because they are inconsistent with them.
➤ Latent narratives lie dormant, to be activated now and then.
➤ Emergent narratives are new ones, just starting to be told.

The case example of Browntown is taken from research of Cheers et al. (2004)

SUMMARY

The interactional perspective of community, with its focus on interactions as the essential quality of community, provides the conceptual framework to understand how communities function. This chapter discussed three understandings of community— a community of place, a common interest community, and a community as a social system. From an interactional perspective, a community of place is a commonly agreed locality where people live and interact within a local society that is make up of organisations, structures, and networks. Social interactions occur in everyday life as residents meet their business and social needs, and these interactions are the essence of community.

The chapter introduced a concept of a community of interest as people who share a consistent set of interactions around a common interest, whether it be an economic, social, political, spiritual, or cultural interest. A community can also be viewed as a social system that is composed of units such as organisations and services. Between these units there are predictable, patterned interactions that persist through time. Finally, there is an evidence-based definition of community for public health practice that stresses the three elements that are in most definitions of community— interactions, a commonly agreed-upon geographic area, and common interests.

The elements of community structure and functioning discussed in the chapter were: the local society; the community field; community power structures; horizontal and vertical patterns of interaction; strong and weak ties; and community narratives. Community health and social care development is most effective when the question, 'What is the community I am working with and how does it function?' can be answered.

USEFUL WEBSITES

The Australian government website for community development information:
> http://www.community.gov.au/

The Sustainable Communities Network for information about community action:
> http://www.sustainable.org/

The Community Development Exchange: http://www.cdx.org.uk/resources/
> strategicframework.htm

Social capital

The Australian government website for information about social capital: http://
> www.community.gov.au/Internet/MFMC/Community.nsf/pages/section?ope
> ndocument&Section=Building%20Social%20Capital

The Australian Bureau of Statistics information about social capital
> research: http://www.abs.gov.au/Websitedbs/c311215.nsf/0/
> 3af45bbd431a127bca256c22007d75ba?OpenDocument

CHAPTER 3

Community: Aboriginal Australian Perspectives

Introduction

This chapter is written by Aboriginal Australians Rachel Cummins, Ian Gentle, and Charmaine Hull.

After outlining recent statistics regarding the health and wellbeing of Aboriginal and Torres Strait Islander people, the authors show that the mainstream construction of Aboriginal community fails to grasp how Aboriginal society works. They then explore how community might better be understood in the context of Aboriginal social life.

In the second half of this chapter, the focus is on helping people to work in partnership with Aboriginal and Torres Strait Islander people.

Rachel's writing is drawn from her learning as a child, and her understanding and experience as an adult. She offers her interpretation of her people's knowledge of their cultural, social, physical and spiritual environment—the Aboriginal wisdom. Rachel has worked in various community services over a number of years, and continues her attempts to meld Aboriginal wisdom into the mainstream agenda.

Charmaine wishes to acknowledge her mother, an Adnyamathanha woman, and her father, an Arabunna and Yankuntjatjara man. Charmaine's experiences in living in Aboriginal communities and the wider community have given her this angle on community. She believes that her education has helped her reflect on the meaning of community as intertwined elements of land, mother-earth, kinship, relationships, responsibilities, and obligation.

Ian tells us about himself:

I am a Nyoongar man of the Upper Swan Reach and after growing up in the city I moved regularly around the mid-west of Western Australia. When I moved to the Northern Territory I experienced Aboriginal community life in both a semi-urban and a traditional sense. Then, when I moved to South Australia, I was able to connect with a specific cultural group which taught me to understand the importance of yourself and who you are. I am now in my homeland in Western Australia after a twenty-five-year cycle working and understanding more about my Nyoongar heritage.

Aboriginal health and wellbeing

It is clearly apparent from a cursory glance at the statistics and health status indicators of Aboriginal and Torres Strait Islander health and wellbeing that there are serious inequities between Indigenous Australians[1] and non-Indigenous populations in Australia. In the period 1999–2001, using current methodology, the life expectancy at birth for Indigenous Australians was estimated to be 56 for males and 63 for females. In contrast, life expectancy for all Australians was 77 for males and 83 for females (Trewin and Madden 2003, p. 182).

It was estimated in 2001 that 2.4 per cent of the Australian population was made up of Indigenous Australians, and at that time less than 32 per cent of households with Indigenous person(s) were home owners compared with 69 per cent for non-Indigenous households (Trewin and Madden 2003, p. 2). At the same time (2001), aggregated data from most Australian states and territories revealed that 34 per cent of juveniles between 10 and 17 years in remand centres were Indigenous Australians (Trewin and Madden 2003, p. 5).

The message from Aboriginal and Torres Strait Islander Australians is clear. 'If grassroots members of our communities do not have involvement in, or ownership of, the solutions to their local problems then any proposed remedies are almost certain to fail' (Quartermaine 2003). Therefore, in addressing the determinants of health and wellbeing, and the inequalities that exist between Indigenous and non-Indigenous Australians, Indigenous Australians must be involved at all levels in determining policy and at all stages in the implementation of initiatives.

This chapter explores three perspectives on what the term 'community' means to Aboriginal Australians as a starting point to a better understanding of how to work in partnership to address the determinants of health and wellbeing through community health and social care development. Although we use the term 'community' throughout the book to refer to all types of communities, we do so accepting that many Aboriginal people understand the term differently. It is essential that this is kept in mind when working with Aboriginal communities. Being aware of some of the differences between Western and Aboriginal understandings of community enables discussion to start about the right way to do things, followed by the development of strong partnerships that are based in this shared understanding.

It is not claimed that the perspectives presented here are representative of all Indigenous people. Many Aboriginal and Torres Strait Islander groups may have different understandings. Rather, the presentations are personal perspectives on how these people have struggled to 'find a way for how community is going to work'.

Non-Indigenous constructions of Aboriginal community

Rachel describes how the term 'community' has been constructed by mainstream society to apply to Aboriginal and Torres Strait Islander communities.

From my perspective, the term 'community' is constructed by non-Indigenous society for a variety of purposes. It is often used to bring together Aboriginal and Torres Strait Islander people as one group. In some cases, to gain funding for a particular program, Aboriginal and Torres Strait Islander people have to present themselves as one community. But if you tease through things, Aboriginal and Torres Strait Islander cultures are very different on a number of levels political, social, and economic and this is obvious in land tenure. One of the reasons Mabo could demonstrate his native title[2] was because Torres Strait Islanders had a system of land title which could be identified and documented.

The current ways that community is constructed for Aboriginal people is so far removed from my knowledge of what Aboriginal community means that I have now to find a way for how these things are going to work. For example, there was a proposal to bring the youth who were having difficulties from the North down to our community here. The idea was that our people and our Elders would talk to them and work with them in building knowledge and identity. But our Elders are saying to us, we can't talk to them about our business; it's not that we don't want to share our business, but it is not proper that we do it. This is because they've got their own business, and in fact we could be insulting their Elders by teaching the young ones our business.

Failure to understand how Aboriginal society works

As we design programs and keep calling things 'the Indigenous community', we are doing a disservice to the Torres Strait Islander and to the Aboriginal communities. There are some people who say, 'Well, we're all one', and of course we are one people with the right to expect housing, education, and everything else. But how these things are delivered, and what makes it work in one community as opposed to another, all comes down to those particular values in those individual communities that are very different.

For as long as we have the statistics that we have—higher levels of incarceration, appalling health status, relatively high drop-out rates in education, a relatively high suicide rate, and child protection issues—I think we need to find out properly what works in individual communities and start from there.

An Aboriginal concept of community

Rachel explains an Aboriginal concept of community.

Aboriginal family relationships are at the core of an Aboriginal interpretation of 'community', and the family relationship or kinship system is not necessarily confined to a geographic territory. The strength of this is that the system is not reliant only on blood ties, but draws on spiritual connections to country and to people. This connection is not weakened by distance.

Aboriginal community is about relationships. This is so important. Aboriginal people connect through the kinship system. It's not only a blood line, it is also about those particular levels of responsibility. Family relationship gives you a particular place within the extended kinship, but it also gives you your totem, and then who your totem is also gives you that responsibility. And your totem tells you the responsibility you have to country.

And so it's not just land care or making sure that the waterways are clean, but it is all connected to the spirituality too. If you don't do particular things, then when you die you won't have a restful time. People are guaranteeing not only their existence but also their peace in the everlasting world. Some of this is getting a bit lost with the loss of our Elders, but when I go back up to my country I know that there are people still there who know these things.

The principle of everyone having a place

In Aboriginal society, every Aboriginal person has a place. Mind you, not everybody knows it, because you have people who have come from the stolen generation,[3] who are still finding their way home. There are people who have been denied their Aboriginality for many reasons. But once people find their way home, there is a place for them. This is because our history was oral, so information about relationships is passed on in this way. For example, my grandfather was removed from his country and family at a young age. However, there are people in their eighties who live in that country who still remember him and his place and they know me and what my place is. Thankfully, in some patches there is still information about family that is passed on, and there are people who are able to tell people where they fit.

That personal relationship and having a place is so important. I was at a community meeting helping to develop services some time ago and one of the older women who came along said, 'We want you to find out where our kids are.' So we said, 'Who are these children?' thinking that we would get one or two names from maybe three or six months ago. But these people mentioned eight children, some of whom had been missing for about twenty years. And of course we couldn't find them, but the community still remembered, the community still had that loss of years ago.

Many aboriginal people still understand themselves as connected in some way. If, for some reason, we have a person who is outside of that, then we will allocate that person a place and put the person in it and say, 'Now you can call me Grandfather, or I can be your grandson.'

For someone to be accepted into our community, we have to find a spot for the person. For example, if a non-Indigenous person new to the community wanted to be accepted into the community then they would have to be assigned a place. A lot of people have come into our community and some have gone away saying, 'Well, I was adopted and I got a skin name and now I know everything tribal'; but this is not correct. It is not really about giving that person information. It's about giving that person a place so that our people know who you are and where you sit and what responsibilities and rights that place gives you. And that's why in the protection of children, in health and wellbeing, in domestic violence, in land, in looking after waterways, it is important to understand what the person's particular place is, because that gives you the particular task.

Culture community

My knowledge of Aboriginal community from the past doesn't work now because of the way Aboriginal social life is now constructed as one 'community'. We have had to struggle hard to find a way that our understanding of Aboriginal community can fit within current service delivery systems. With my non-Aboriginal colleague Tricia Hays, we decided to use the term 'culture community'.

A culture community, unlike the concept of a community of place, discussed in the previous chapter, has no geographic boundaries. It is made up of those people who connect because of kinship and culture, wherever their location. This means that in a 'historical' community, made up of people from different kinship networks who have been relocated by mainstream society to a geographic area, there may be different culture communities. The identification with the culture community may be stronger than the identification with the historical community.

The implications of this are that an Aboriginal person may be part of many communities, but if there is membership of a culture community, this will predominate. I'm part of many communities, including a culture community.

I have connectedness with Traditional Owner Groups[4] here because of kinship lines. This is my culture community. Then I am part of the Aboriginal community in this town because we are all Aboriginal people and there is automatically a relationship. Then there is my historical community that I am part of because of coming from the same place and a shared history. Then as individuals we belong to other groups and communities, such as a women's group. But there are many Aboriginal people in this town who are still trying to find their way into a community. They know they have a place, and they are told that they have a place, but they can't feel or experience it. They are lost.

Conflicts around perceptions of community

There are many examples where Indigenous and non-Indigenous perspectives on community conflict. These concern family structure and responsibilities. A term that I struggle with is the non-Indigenous use of the term 'extended family' to explain Aboriginal family relationships. When I was growing up, I had eight or nine mothers and grandmothers and all of that, and so I took it for granted that all these people had different responsibilities to the children. That's how we grew up. But when I went away from my home I had to learn a whole new language.

I am not comfortable with the term 'extended family' to describe my kinship connections. I would be talking and I would say 'my brother'. People would look at me strangely and say, 'I didn't know you had a brother—oh you mean your cousin', and I felt like I betrayed my kinship connections by saying 'cousin' because that term is too foreign, too removed. So I tried the term 'cousin brother', because I didn't feel comfortable saying 'cousin'.

Sometimes at work, my family would come in and leave messages for me, like 'Oh, just say her brother was here'. Of course the receptionist just takes the message, and doesn't ask any further for the person's name. When I get the message, I don't know who it is. It could be anybody who is my brother. The receptionist replies, 'But surely you must know who your brother is.'

Another point is that Aboriginal society, contrary to common belief, was very structured and ordered. For example, protocols are very strict and enforced with regard to land, law, and social obligations. However, some of the clarity around these structures has been disrupted in us by trying to fit into this other non-Indigenous community.

There are different responsibilities for family members. The grandparents' responsibility to children was to inform them, at the right time, all about marital relationships and responsibilities. Then, depending on the kinship structure, all the mothers and fathers and the aunties and uncles have a particular nurturing responsibility. With the demise of family, children sometimes don't get the information or the nurturing they need because the aunty, uncle, or grandparent who had that responsibility couldn't talk to them, was too old, or burdened.

These roles and responsibilities are all tied up in how the community functions. If the roles and responsibilities are not intact, then community is not able to function. If people are broken away from that kinship structure in some way through the stolen generation and there are missing links, then that sense of loss makes it difficult for people to get back and actually know their links. Maybe they have been told that they have a place, but they have no way of really knowing it. They remain without a feeling of connectedness. Here is an example of the interconnections there are between land, kinship, and responsibilities.

CASE EXAMPLE 3.1

Interconnections between kinship, responsibilities, and land: A Traditional Owner organisation

Traditional Owners Groups are kinship groups that express native title rights and a custodian relationship with the land that they come from. In northern Queensland, nine Traditional Owner Groups have joined together to become an incorporated organisation, which gives the groups the means to apply for funding for programs.

The groups consider that land and community business are all intertwined and that 'you can't care for people if you don't care for country'. One Traditional Owner explains the connections between land, kinship, and responsibilities and why it is important to get 'back on country'.

There are a lot of problems with domestic violence and other problems and it is important for people to get back on country. Some of our children are getting into trouble and they should be coming here to our land and our old people should be teaching them. If you give them a bit more pride, then they won't be doing those things. It is strength for those children to know who they are. In knowing their country, they know their responsibility and they know where they fit in their Aboriginal world. Although we know that there is a dilemma in coming outside of their country and coming into our Western system, we must help our children know their ways.

Think about it

➤ How are land business and community business intertwined?

➤ What do you think are the dilemmas for young people fitting into Aboriginal ways while being part of the mainstream education and employment systems?

➤ Do you think Aboriginal people would experience problems if they don't know their place?

Charmaine Hull, an Adnyamathanha women from the Flinders Ranges in South Australia discusses her understanding of what community means.

I don't really use the word 'community'. As Aboriginal people, you either associate with the Aboriginal tribal group you come from or you associate with the land that you come from. So the term 'community' isn't something that we use as Aboriginal people. When I am away from home, people don't ask me what community I come from; they ask me, 'What land do you come from, which area, where do you belong, and who are your people?' I guess the word 'community' is alien to Aboriginal people.

For us it is not just infrastructure and buildings, it is about us as people as individuals and the larger group. The larger group may cover quite a large area. For example some Adnyamathanha people may live together in a town, but the community would extend further up because you've got family living within the Adnyamathanha area and that is also considered as community.

History has got a lot to do with a lot of people feeling dispossessed and not being part of their land. Unfortunately, in cities Aboriginal people can't go back to the significant sites, as a lot of areas have been bulldozed. We can't knock the buildings down and put it back the way it was. Aboriginal people who live within cities know that they are the custodians of that area but they are unable to visit important sites because there are freeways, houses, and new developments coming up. What can the people do? This is destroying the soul of Aboriginal people.

Then there is the way that Aboriginal people were removed from their land, through various forms. Many Aboriginal people did not return to their family. So you just have to look at history and that's why there are a lot of issues today around communities, obligation, and law and order, and all these sorts of things. So history has got a lot to do with it.

Ian Gentle describes his understanding of place and the difference between a place and a town. He finds the term 'place' more meaningful than the term 'community'.

I understand community as people who belong to each other and to a common place. The place may be spread over a vast area. For example, for the people living in Port Augusta, their community includes people in Coober Pedy right throughout Marree and Leigh Creek. It is important for me to understand how people fit within their place. We focus on people and place rather than on the specific town in which people live. This is because historically Aboriginal people were moved away from their traditional areas, sometimes forcibly,[5] and were made to go to missions, reserves and townships in settled areas. The places where people have been brought to may not have been part of their traditional area, but a place where they have to stay to gain employment or education. While these people may live in this town they still retain ties to other places.

I think there needs to be another term for what is termed the Aboriginal 'community'. What has happened is that over the last three generations we have had to use the term 'community' to identify with a specific location in order to get services. Therefore it has become the pattern to refer to an Aboriginal community as a specific town where a group of people live and work. People say, 'Oh, but why do you travel from here to here? We can't keep track of you all the time.' But we say, 'Well hang on, this is where I come from. This town is only the place where I go to get services; where I live is out here in the bush, in the place.'

The Aboriginal names for places reflect the whole area, not just the town. An example of this is the name 'Uluru'.[6] This refers to the whole place that surrounds the rock. The non-Indigenous use of the term 'Ayres Rock' simply referred to the rock. We have ways of knowing and understanding that it is really place, not simply a town, or a specific geographical feature, that is important to us.

We have got all the homeland programs in an area now because people don't belong to one place, they belong to many places. Boundaries may overlap in a number of places because people are related. Arabuna people are related to Adnyamathanha, and Adnyamathanha people are related to Kukatja people, and it all just makes up one large 'community'.

Ian describes how each Aboriginal person has a place and the importance of finding a place, and how, in his case, this took a long time.

I have travelled halfway around this country trying to find my place. I have lived in many different places, but now finding my place is really important. I have lived in South Australia and even though I was adopted very well into this place, with my family and the Nepabunna and Arabuna community accepting me in, it wasn't until I went home back to Perth that I actually found my place, and I had to stand there at the Swan River with my uncle and he showed me all these places that I have been travelling for many years trying to find. This doesn't mean that Port Augusta is no longer my place, but now I have found something else that I've been looking for all my life. This place is who I am and who I'm going to be, and that's really good.

When I grew up as a child in a big city, I found that there was nothing, that there was no connection. You were told your connections were taken away from you back through the processes of being removed from your country, being put in missions or reserves and being told you're not allowed to do that any more [to speak language and practise culture].

A lot of people who have lived in the city all their life don't know who they are and they've never been able to reconnect with their family or their community. This turns into chaos for groups of people and leads to some of the issues for us today. For example, back in those early days, the role of the men was taken away from them, so they weren't living any more the cultural ways.

Ian describes some of the effects of the loss of connection to place.

One of the consequences of this loss of role is that men began to perpetrate crimes that weren't part of the Aboriginal culture, and this is very evident today. Related to this are the health problems, and many Aboriginal men are dying before they're fifty. Then there is no father to bring up the children in the way in which it should be done, so young people are not told their place.

A lot of Aboriginal people don't know where their place is, but one day they will find it and when they do the 'coin will drop' and you will know where you are inside. Our people have studied the universe for a long, long time and our universe is set on the sun and that is the place of significance and everything rotates around the sun. So, in Aboriginal ways, the sun is the place. The Earth, the Moon, Jupiter, and Mars all rotate around the sun; and when Aboriginal people don't have a sense of place or where they come from, they circle around like the planets. They are always part of the loop but they are not sure where their place is.

We are starting to build a place for our young people now, but it's going to take another two or three generations and we really need to go back a couple of steps. This is still only the first and second generation since Aboriginal people were counted and had the right to vote.[7] In 1967, I was deemed an Australian citizen; but before that, I was part of the natural flora and fauna, so how could we understand where community is? Back then, we weren't part of the bigger scheme of things.

Ian explains what is meant by 'obligation'.

Our obligation is not only to the living but also to the gone; the people who are not here any more. The fact is that you may have to travel 3000 kilometres from a place to another place to have a funeral; and you need to do that because of the obligation to the family, and to the person; and you have got to fulfil that obligation, otherwise you will forever feel empty for not doing that. Sometimes, people who bring their whole families down for a funeral have never met the person who has passed on. The kids didn't even know they had this relative, but the mother or father know their people and you have to pay respect. This is the obligation that we are talking about.

Charmaine talks about how it is impossible to separate the elements land, mother-earth, kinship, relationships, responsibilities, and obligation.

As they say, from the creation of the Dreamtime,[8] you have the land, mother-earth, and you have the people, and you can't separate these elements. I understand that the Aboriginal community is based on kinship, relationships, responsibilities, and obligation. I guess the obligation falls in line with who we are within the family, those kinship relationships within a particular family, and so you know you do have obligations that have been set in place. You can't separate the people from the land because we also have an obligation to the land and caring for the land, so that's why you can't separate the two.

The knowledge about responsibilities and obligation has been passed down through time so every Aboriginal person has an obligation to the family and that includes community as well because community is made up of that kinship. Kinship makes up community and this includes particular groups, for example Adnyamathanha, and the people that marry someone from that group. That marriage brings them into that community.

Summary

The first half of this chapter explored how three Aboriginal Australians understand 'community'. Overall, they would prefer not to use the term, because it does not really explain the importance of kinship, relationships, responsibilities, and obligations that are fundamental to Aboriginal social life. However, the term 'community' is going to continue to be used in Aboriginal and Indigenous contexts, so the following points are important.

Practice tip 3.1

➤ The term 'Indigenous community' is most often used to refer to Indigenous people living in a town—for example, the 'Port Augusta Aboriginal community'. In Port Augusta, there are different kinship groups; and people move to and from their land to fulfil their responsibilities and obligations. These groups may or may not be able to be described as one 'community'.

➤ Aboriginal people may belong to more than one community. There may be membership of a 'culture community', a Traditional Owner Group, an Aboriginal community in a town, and other communities of interest.

➤ All Aboriginal people have a place in kinship structures. Some Aboriginal people are finding their place. Having a place is about having responsibilities and obligations to land and to family. It is impossible to separate out these elements.

Activity 3.1

Key elements of an Aboriginal understanding of community

Can you summarise in your own words what are the key components of an Aboriginal understanding of community?

Why do you think it is important to understand how Indigenous people understand the term 'community'?

Working with Aboriginal communities

The second half of this chapter is written in order to help people work in equivalent intercultural partnerships (Franks et al., 2007) with Aboriginal communities, families, organisations, and individuals in community health and social care development.

Rachel describes how important it is to find a new way of working with Aboriginal communities.

In the past we have often extended programs to Aboriginal and Torres Strait Islander people by 'putting a black face' on promotion material, and considered that to be enough.

The current models of service delivery are not always working, and it is not about money. You can put in a million dollars, and a million dollars on top of that, but if the model is not right and the people don't feel that they have a say in determining and developing and not just running the model after it happens, it won't work. People have to have a say in determining and developing the models.

We need to acknowledge the way that Aboriginal communities want to do business, and we are struggling to do this. One model, promoted by Traditional Owner Groups in North Queensland, is a model of service provision based on the culture community.

It involves bringing people to their land, and 'a whole mob of our lot' go out and spend weeks with them; not just with mum and dad who have issues, and not just with dad and son, who might have issues. It means bringing a whole culture community together with Elders and intertwining teachings around domestic violence and, as well, people's responsibilities to the country, the water, the trees, the animals, and learning from that. But this approach doesn't fit with current

Activity 3.2

Enabling groups to provide integrated services and initiatives

Government agencies rarely fund programs that enable groups to take care of all the aspects of community life. Usually programs are for particular target groups, such as young people at risk of becoming involved in the justice system or for women experiencing domestic violence.

Returning to Case example 3.1, it is clear that the Traditional Owner Organ-isation would like to provide services for their young people by getting them back to country in order that they can learn more about their Aboriginal world.

Think about it

➤ Why does the Traditional Owner Organisation want to take care of providing services for its young people?

➤ What are some the ways for practitioners to work with the Traditional Owner Group to help enable these services to commence?

funding options; and therefore, the groups concerned must move their ideas into ways that are consistent with government programs. Activity 3.2 (page 55) shows how difficult it is to match needs to funding opportunities.

Practice tip 3.2

➤ Always approach charitable trusts and philanthropic organisations to seek funding that can be used flexibly.
➤ Don't make assumptions about the structure of an Aboriginal community. You need to find an appropriate way to ask questions.

Charmaine talks about why it is important to tread carefully in working with communities.

I think the important thing when you first go to a community is to speak to the Elders and Custodians of that area. I think the other thing is remembering that in some communities there are divisions among groups. We have to be realistic about this and find out what those divisions are. We find out about those divisions from talking to service providers as, generally, they cannot be biased towards any group.

Service providers will tell you if it's OK if you go and speak to Uncle Joe over here as he's with this group and if you go and talk with Uncle Ben when he's with this other group. It is important that you go and speak to both groups. In some communities there may be three different groups, so you have to have three different meetings. It is essential that you speak to everybody and not just one group.

It is important to remember that you have to build that rapport, particularly with the key people. To do this you need to go and talk among the people before the meeting or event that you are planning. The other thing is going back to the community and validating what you think people were saying. You may need to show people the notes that you took—'This is what I've written and what do you think about it?'

People have a habit of going out and getting a story, and then they are gone with what they believe is a wonderful story. Sometimes, though, it is not true or correct, because the person didn't go back to validate it. This can create a barrier between you and the community or it can create further friction between groups where there is already a division. It is important not to always believe that everything's rosy and that it is all 'one community'. It is not always like that. So you have to tread really carefully.

As people coming in to work with a community, you need to make it very clear that you're there as a neutral person and that you are there for everyone. One of the biggest problems with people when they come in and work is that they align themselves with one particular group and then it creates a division straight away.

When I go into a community that is not my country, I really need to do my homework and find out who are the Traditional Custodians of the country? Then I need to know where the divisions are and if there is a 'tug of war' going on. Then I need to speak with all these different groups in order to work properly. I know it is important not to rush things, because if you do you are not going to get the outcome that you expected. Timing is crucial as well.

Practice tip 3.3

Timing is a really important issue. Rarely is it the case that practitioner's timeframes and community's will coincide. Every situation is different and it must be carefully negotiated.

Activity 3.3

A family violence prevention initiative

In Case example 3.1, a Traditional Owner Organisation made up of nine Traditional Owner Groups was described. The Organisation has a chairperson, a management committee, and a community development worker is employed. If you would like to talk to this organisation about family violence prevention strategies, whom would you approach and why?

Charmaine describes why it is important to sit down with people and understand where they are coming from.

People working with communities need to come and sit down and do what Fred Hollows did—sit with the people for days and days on end, and sit in their environment to understand it. It is not possible to get a full understanding if you don't go through that process. You need to live that life to really understand where people have come from and where they're going to. So a lot of work needs to be done in that area and it's not going to happen overnight. A lot of healing needs to be done as well for people to move on. We need as Aboriginal people to nurture our culture before it is lost. Elders are actually passing on with a lot of that knowledge and information, and our young people are being swallowed up by the Western culture.

Charmaine explains how exposure to two different systems of knowledge, culture, and spirituality has caused confusion among Aboriginal people.

It is the two cultures clashing. It's a cultural clash for a lot of our children. On the one hand, we're telling our children to get a good education because we want our children to succeed. However, because we are supporting good education, our children are getting caught up in this Western culture. It is inevitable that there will be a lot of confusion among our children because of the exposure to very different systems of knowledge, culture, and spirituality. It is especially our children, the next generation, who are finding it hard. We tell them that it is essential to get a good education in order to go to university, get a good job to have enough money to buy a house and a car. Then, on the other hand, we tell them to come up with us to feel our country. There's just so much for them to take in, so there's a lot of confusion.

The history has caused a lot of confusion of us as Aboriginal people. At one time we are being removed from our culture. We are being told we need to integrate but then we are segregated. The 'welfare mentality'[9] came in at a time when Aboriginal people were very vulnerable and being removed from country.

I think what needs to happen is that government needs to go down and really sit down with Aboriginal people and say 'well what it is it that you want?' That's only been happening for a very short period. It hasn't happened in the past as we've been told what to do and when to do it. Change happens at a very slow pace and we're not going to see results and outcomes until two, three, or four generations down the track.

Ian talks about what is important in working with communities.

I think what we need to do first is really find out and talk to some of the leaders in the community—the Custodians, the people who have the knowledge. We need to really find out what is the history of the place, how do you work with the community, who are the main players in the group, and to get the OK from them on how to do things, and ask people exactly what they really want, not what we think they need or want, but what do they really want.

The ways in which Aboriginal groups function are outside the Western paradigm, and administrators fail to see the fact that they are doing things incorrectly by talking to the wrong people, or missing important people.

Unfortunately, in the past, too many people have just gone into a community and said, 'I think this is a great idea; we'll do this for you.' Three years down the line, there would be nothing there that the people used. The project became a white elephant; now how many white elephants are there in Aboriginal communities around this country? There are hundreds of them, thousands.

Sometimes the more outspoken person of the community might not be the right person to talk to. I always use the analogy of driving into a community and you see three people. You see the old fellow who sits in a little humpy just outside the community and you pass by him. Then you see the old lady sitting on the other side over there and you pass by her. Then you go over and talk to the community development officer and you ask him your questions. He will give you his perspective, but he will say, 'Go back and talk to that person you passed by on the way in, because he is an Elder and you need to talk with him.'

The community council is sometimes made up of a lot of people across the whole spectrum, and sometimes there are factions within the council. These factions may be along family lines because the relationships between families have been eroded. Before, it was a sharing environment, and now that's changed and it is about getting what we can for our survival. This is not because I want to be greedy, but because I need to survive and I need to provide for my children.

Notes

1 Indigenous Australian refers to those Australians of Aboriginal and Torres Strait Islander descent.

2 In 1992, the assumption of *terra nullius* was struck down by the Australian High Court in the Mabo decision, which granted Mer (Murray Island) in the Torres Strait to the Meriam people. Justice Brennan stated in *Mabo (No. 2)*, 'Native title has its origin and is given its content by the traditional laws acknowledged by and the customs observed by the Indigenous inhabitants of a territory.' See also, *Native Title Act 1993* (Cth).

3 The stolen generation refers to all those Aboriginal children who were forcibly removed and stolen from their families by Australian state and territory authorities in order to be assimilated into mainstream culture. These children were placed in church missions, orphanages, institutions, or employment where they lost contact with their families and their culture.

4 Traditional Owner Groups are kinship groups that express native title rights and a custodian relationship with the land that they come from. Sometimes these groups have formal structures and may be formally incorporated.

5 Forcible removal of Aboriginal people from their place occurred when people were imprisoned, or 'resettled' when the land was mined, or children were stolen from their families, or when whole families were moved to reserves on the fringes of towns.

6 Uluru in Central Australia is an area of special significance to Aboriginal people.

7 In 1967, a national referendum was conducted in Australia, which determined that Indigenous people should be part of the national census and given the right to vote.

8 Dreamtime is most often used to describe the 'time before time', or 'the time of the creation of all things', while 'Dreaming' is often used to refer to an individual's or group's set of beliefs or spirituality.

9 A 'welfare mentality' is an expectation that government will or should provide resources for people to live.

SUMMARY

This chapter provided a framework in which to understand the importance of the family relationship or kinship system to Aboriginal people and their spiritual connections to country. This understanding is fundamental to working with Aboriginal people, organisations, and communities. Partnerships based in this shared understanding will assist people in working in community health and social care development.

The important points are:

➤ Understand the Aboriginal community you are working with, and know who are the Custodians and the important people.
➤ Take time to find out the history of the community, and when you first go to a community speak to the Elders and Custodians of that area to build relationships.
➤ Talk among the people before the meeting or event that you are planning.
➤ Go back to the community and validate what you thought people were saying.
➤ Understand the differences among groups and organisations.

USEFUL WEBSITES

The Foundation for Aboriginal and Torres Strait Islander Research Action is a community-based Indigenous rights organisation: http://www.faira.org.au/
The Australian Human Rights and Equal Opportunities Commission; Aboriginal and Torres Strait Islander social justice home page: http://www.humanrights.gov.au/social_justice/stolen_children/index.html
The National Centre for Aboriginal and Torres Strait Islander Statistics: http://www.abs.gov.au/Websitedbs/c311215.nsf/0/7b42698ca2264d4bca256e540071b1d9?OpenDocument

Indigenous health

The Australian Department of Health and Ageing's site on Indigenous Health: http://www.health.gov.au/internet/wcms/publishing.nsf/Content/Indigenous+Health-1lp
For information about Indigenous health: http://www.healthinfonet.ecu.edu.au/

CHAPTER 4

Community Capacity

Introduction

This chapter aims to:

➤ explain the concepts that help us understand community capacity-including community strength, entrepreneurial social infrastructure, and social capital;
➤ define community capacity; and
➤ enable practitioners and communities to assess community capacity.

The chapter focuses on a community's social capacities to enhance individual and collective health and wellbeing, engage in social and economic development, and solve local problems. We discuss what community capacity is, what we know about it, and how to measure it. Community capacities include, for example, leadership skills, social structures such as clubs, hospitals, and community organisations, and how people organise their relations with each other and the outside world to get things done. Without a clear understanding of a community's capacities, the practitioner will find it hard to use them and to help others to use them. Although much of what we know about community capacity comes from research on communities of place, the concept applies equally well to communities of interest.

We also discuss some related concepts that deepen our understanding of community capacity. These include community strength (Black and Hughes 2001; Cheers et al. 2004), entrepreneurial social infrastructure (Flora 1998), and social capital (Bourdieu 1985; Coleman 1988; Portes 1998; Putnam 1995). Case example 4.1 (page 62) is an example of some of the capacities available to people in a community of place to support various types of development.

CASE EXAMPLE 4.1

Yellowleaf's community capacities

In Australia, keeping health and community services in regional communities is of the utmost importance. At the community level, there is no debate about the connection of viable and relevant health and community services with economic and social sustainability. The ability to access a comprehensive range of health and human services attracts newcomers to take up local employment opportunities, encourages older people to stay, and increases everyone's feelings of security. Local services also provide employment opportunities. Generally, threats to reduce service levels, withdraw hospital beds, and relocate services to larger centres attract community outcry and predictions of community decline, demonstrating that health and human services have a wider role in the community beyond service provision.

Some communities take a proactive role in keeping services viable. Yellowleaf is one of these. With a regional population of 50,000, Yellowleaf is the centre for local government and has a diverse industrial base. Over the years, community members have contributed financially to maintaining health services, the cultural centre, and sporting and service clubs. They were actively involved in reconfiguring the health services when it was difficult to attract and retain doctors. When several of the town's banks were closed in the 1990s, the community decided that the withdrawal of banking services may compromise the longer-term prosperity of the town. So they established a community-sponsored bank.

Employment is available for most people in Yellowleaf because of emerging industries. For instance, a group of people with refugee status recently settled in the town because of local employment opportunities. Other members of the community are bringing these newcomers into the life of the town by including them in community activities and modifying facilities and services so they are more appropriate to them. For example, a weekly 'women-only' swimming session was introduced to the local pool especially for Muslim women, and a cultural group enabling the community to understand more about Islam meets regularly.

Community leaders in local government are represented on the management boards of the hospital, health services, and service clubs. Most people regard the community as relatively affluent, pro-development, and go-ahead. Nevertheless, older residents see that things are changing.

While they recognise that the long-time community leaders are working on behalf of the community, they are perturbed that young people are not contributing, and concerned that community spirit, demonstrated by a life-long commitment to volunteering, is diminishing. They are uncertain about whether the newcomers, especially those with different cultural and ethnic backgrounds, can understand the need for the community to work together to maintain the level of services that people expect. These older adults see that it is the same people who continue to take on leadership positions, frequently several at a time.

The 'community factor'

The Yellowleaf community described in Case example 4.1 has been able to bring together its financial resources and human skills to develop its industries and maintain its community and health services, sporting facilities, and service clubs. It has an active and inclusive community field linking the activities of various social fields. At the level of community field, as discussed in Chapter 2 (see also Wilkinson 1970, 1991), people interact with their shared physical and social structures and resources to coordinate activities across social fields to develop the community socially and economically. Communities vary from one another and over time in their success at doing this. Many factors contribute to this diversity, including the community's natural environment, economic potential, investment in physical infrastructure such as roads and buildings, geographic location, service infrastructure, individual skills, and sheer chance (Wilkinson 1972, p. 45).

However, these variables do not fully explain differences between communities with respect to their capacity to support health and human services, social development, education, economic development, and so on. There is also a community-level factor at work. Coming from different assumptions and theoretical frameworks, there have been many attempts to define and measure the 'community factor'. Concepts such as 'community strength', 'community capacity', 'social capital', 'community resiliency', 'social cohesion', 'community activeness', and 'community efficacy' have been used (Cheers et al. 2004).

We define the community factor as all the capacities a community has that are inherent in how it functions socially. For instance, individual skills become community capacities and contribute to total community wellbeing only when they are engaged for the community's benefit through social interaction. This happens, for example, when someone from the community health centre engages a person with the required expertise for a particular task.

Black and Hughes (2001, p. 3) distinguish between 'hard' and 'soft' capacities. 'Hard capacities' include, for example, the physical and material infrastructure, such as meeting rooms, information technology, financial resources, and the like, and may be 'social' or 'private'. 'Social' capacities are owned and maintained by the community generally, or made available to it through processes that involve social interaction. In contrast, 'private' capacities can only be accessed by particular individuals and businesses. For example, while the general practitioner might own the medical equipment and facilities in a surgery, such as computers and fax machines, the surgery building itself is a community capacity because it is owned and maintained by the community generally.

'Soft' capacities are relational ones including, for example, traditions of volunteering, patterns of local social interaction, such as the strong and weak ties discussed in Chapter 2 (Granovetter 1973), qualities of relations, such as social capital, leadership patterns, shared attitudes and values, and individual skills as they are made available to the community generally. As we shall see later in this chapter, 'soft' capacities, too, can be defined, measured, profiled, and developed.

Activity 4.1

Types of capacities

What are some of the 'hard capacities' that Yellowleaf has?
What are some of the 'soft capacities' that Yellowleaf has?

Are community capacities generic or purpose-specific?

There is ongoing debate about whether community capacity is generic or varies according to the purpose at hand. Are, for example, the capacities required to support a nutrition education program based at the local high schools identical to those needed to support the development and maintenance of a community-owned bank?

Given that primary health care and community development share some common elements (Foster 1982, p. 184), it is not surprising that community capacities identified in the health promotion literature (Goodman 1998 et al.) are similar to those considered necessary for community development (Cheers and Luloff 2001). For instance, Goodman et al. (1998, p. 260) described what they called the dimensions of community capacity that are central to communities effectively engaging in health promotion as community participation and leadership, skills and resources relevant to health promotion, and social and inter-organisational networks, a sense of community, and an understanding of community history. Similarly, writing about community development, Cheers et al. (2007) identified capacities such as leadership, social infrastructure resources (e.g. clubs and community development organisations), networks and partnerships between individuals and organisations, and community heritage narratives.

Nevertheless, although there is clearly overlap, health promotion researchers tend to emphasise organisational and individual capacities, while community development researchers focus more on community-level ones. For instance, after surveying health promotion practitioners and leaders of regional health care organisations, McLean et al. (2001, p. 257) grouped organisational and individual capacities into knowledge, skills, commitments, and resources required by individuals and organisations to effectively plan, implement, and evaluate health promotion activities.

Cheers, Kruger, and Trigg's (2005) pilot research on community capacity to support the development of primary industries identified sixteen capacities. However, this work was later modified by Hylton Keele and Cosgrove in 2007 to produce a broader-based template with seventeen capacities. These included both organisational factors, such as programs and facilities, as well as community-level relational factors, such as leadership and advocacy.

Whereas respondents to McLean et al. focused on selected capacities to support health promotion, Cheers, Kruger and Trigg's (2005) participants regarded all the sixteen capacities as essential to all kinds of development, even though the latter project focused specifically on primary industries.

In effect, then, in contrast with McLean et al. (2001, p. 257), Cheers, Kruger, and Trigg (2005) defined community capacity as a generic rather than a purpose-specific construct. Even so, we need more research on this issue and, regardless of whether it is generic or more specific, on the relative importance of various capacities for different kinds of development. Which capacities, for example, are most crucial for supporting the introduction of a communitywide chronic illness prevention program, the development of a youth drop-in centre, and maintaining the local tourism industry?

Furthermore, although research suggests that community capacities in rural communities are generic or, at the very least, overlapping, this finding cannot be transposed to neighbourhoods in urban areas and regional centres without further investigation. Because they are not informed by Indigenous understandings of community and community development, mainstream ideas about community capacity based on Western social science cannot be applied uncritically to Indigenous communities (Chino and DeBruyn 2006).

Practice tip 4.1

Using community capacity assessments with Indigenous communities must be done with care. The understanding of community and how to bring about social cohesion may be different.

Community strength

We choose to use the concept of community strength to describe the community factor. We use this concept because a recent review of the professional literature arrived at a construct that was similar to that of rural participants in a South Australian study (Cheers et al. 2000, 2004). The research participants described 'the community factor' as community strength. All groups—journalists, politicians, primary health care workers, government personnel, service providers, and rural people—agreed that a strong community is good for health, business, social cohesion, managing social issues, and personal wellbeing.

CASE EXAMPLE 4.2

The Enterprise Committee

Source: Cheers et al. 2004, p. 150

> We have a very lively Enterprise Committee in this community and it is this group that sort of ties it [community people engaging with social infrastructure] all together. We have the volunteers who run fundraising events and a retired nurse who runs a weekly exercise group. One of the local men helps us keep the health centre in shape, and we have the Community Enterprise Craft Shop, which gives a percentage of its earnings to community activities. (Rural participant in a South Australian study)

This participant saw people and their organisations in their community engaging with each other and their social infrastructure (skills, networks, and relationships) for the benefit of their community through particular projects, with the Enterprise Committee (the central community field structure) 'tying it all together' or, in other words, organising how they engaged.

In keeping with our definition of 'community' in Chapter 2, and our use of community interaction theory, Cheers and his colleagues (2004) defined community strength as '*people (and their organisations) engaging with each other and their community's social infrastructure for the betterment of the community*'. Case example 4.2 is an example of community strength.

Activity 4.2

Bringing together people and resources in Yellowleaf

Return to Case example 4.1. What are the ways that the Yellowleaf community brings together its people and resources?

Components of community strength

Figure 4.1 presents the components of community strength. It is a dynamic concept, which means that all components are related to one another and it only exists as it happens. In other words, community strength is not something 'out there' waiting to be discovered and activated. It happens spontaneously and is often facilitated by a designated organisation or community worker.

The notion of community betterment focuses community strength on a purpose, whether it is community betterment generally or a particular one such as development of social care services. Black and Hughes (2001, p. 3) make explicit the relationship between community strength and community betterment, when they define community strength as 'the extent to which resources and processes within a community maintain and enhance both individual and collective wellbeing in ways that are consistent with the principles of equity, comprehensiveness, participation, self-relance, and social responsibility'. According to Black and Hughes (2001, p. 4), the qualities of social processes such as trust and trust-worthiness within relationships are just as important to community strength as their quantity.

There are several factors that affect community strength:

➤ the extent to which the community's social relations, interactions, and structures enable engagement with the social infrastructure;

➤ the human resources available to community members, both as individuals and collectively, for such engagement; and

FIGURE 4.1   Community strength

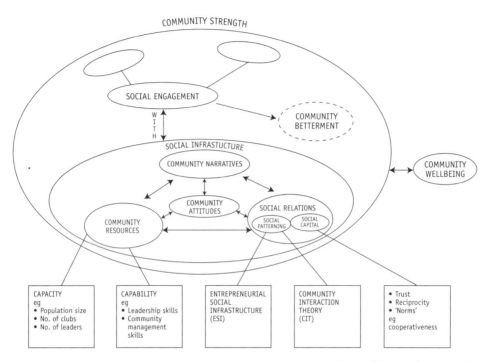

Source: Cheers et al 2004, p. 148

➤ the extent to which they engage the available material, physical, financial, human, and social resources through their social relations, interactions, and structures.

Is community strength always positive?

Whether or not high levels of community strength always have positive outcomes for all community members is debatable (Edwards et al. 2003). Communities that are strongly engaged with their social infrastructure and have the ability to mobilise local people around development projects may do so because of community norms that support participation and cohesiveness. Bernard (1973), for instance, showed that there is a significant positive relationship between cohesiveness and a community's influence on its members to conform. However, those who do not participate in a way that is consistent with the prevailing norms, for whatever reasons, frequently experience exclusion.

At an individual level, a strong community may also engender a 'sense of community'. This happens when people matter to each other, fit together, share some values, and meet their needs through association with one another. This individual experience becomes a community-level phenomenon when it is shared and reinforced through interactions and relations between people. (McMillan and Chavis 1986, p. 13).

Social infrastructure

As Figure 4.1 shows, part of community strength is social infrastructure. Social infrastructure has several components. These are:

➤ community narratives;
➤ community attitudes;
➤ community resources; and
➤ social relations, including social patterning and social capital.

Community narratives

The different types of community narratives were discussed in Chapter 2. They are the stories a community tells about itself. Heritage narratives are passed on down the years, and often contain solutions to past problems that astute leaders can harness to solve present ones. Here is an example that community leaders used to motivate residents to work together to establish a community bank when commercial banking services were withdrawn (Kennedy 2004, p. 80).

CASE EXAMPLE 4.3

A country town's heritage narrative

Many years earlier, the community had saved the town from a major flood by working hard for several days to build 'banks' of sandbags. This story was passed down through the years as the heritage narrative that residents can work hard together to save the town from adversity by building a 'bank'. The current threat to the community's survival involved a major economic downturn and withdrawal of the major banking companies. Community leaders linked this powerful heritage narrative to the present adversity to motivate residents to work together to build another kind of 'bank'.

Activity 4.3

Identifying community narratives

Think of a community of place or of interest that you are familiar with. Can you identify a community narrative that may influence community health or social care development?

Practice tip 4.2

Always check out whether or not community narratives are held across the community.

Community attitudes

Community attitudes are shared views that people in the community have about various issues. For example, in some communities mental health issues are a taboo topic. While people privately may have an understanding and experience of a problem, such as depression, they may be unwilling to acknowledge this publicly. The general view in the community might be that people, if they are down, should 'get over it and get themselves into a decent job'. This attitude, if shared, makes it difficult to engage in effective health promotion.

Activity 4.4

Identifying relevant community attitudes

Using the same community that you are familiar with, can you identify any community attitudes that may influence community health or social care development?

Community resources

Community resources encompass its capacities—individual resources, such as clubs and the skills of individuals—and its capabilities to use these—relational resources, such as leadership and management skills (Cheers et al. 2006). As discussed earlier, capacities and capabilities are not *community* capacities unless people are engaging with them for the benefit of the entire community. We can distinguish between the community resources a community has that might potentially be used for development, and the community's ability to use them for these purposes in changing economic, social, and environmental contexts (Cheers, Kruger, and Trigg 2005, p. 11). Community resources have three defining characteristics:

➤ They are inherent in how the community functions socially, which means that they are owned and/or maintained by people in the community generally.
➤ They contribute to community wellbeing as they are engaged through social interaction.
➤ They are generally available to people and organisations in the community for a variety of purposes, and their use is not restricted to particular individuals, organisations, or enterprises.

Activity 4.5

Identifying community resources

Which of the following are community resources?

➤ The aged person's facility in a city suburb has a ten-seater bus, which can only be driven by an employee of the facility and used by residents of the facility.
➤ The neighbourhood centre has a meeting room available for rent to local groups. The craft group meets there regularly.

Social relations

Social relations, the fourth component of social infrastructure, include:

➤ social patterning, or how the links between people, organisations, and groups are arranged as entrepreneurial social infrastructure; and
➤ the community's social capital.

Social patterning

Some conceptual tools for understanding how social relations are patterned were introduced in Chapter 2. These include horizontal and vertical ties, and strong and weak ties. Communities have various social fields as well as the community field where people work together for the good of the entire community.

Another framework, entrepreneurial social infrastructure (ESI), is relevant to understanding social patterning. ESI emphasises organising social relations into a '...*particular format for developing organizational forms that encourage collective action to achieve tangible goals*' (Flora 1998, p. 489). In other words, ESI answers the question. 'How do people organise their relationships with each other and establish organisational structures to get things done together in an entrepreneurial way?' Activities include, for example, developing and maintaining health services, economic and business development, attracting tourists, or establishing a youth drop-in centre. In Flora's terms, '*a community with a well-developed social infrastructure tends to engage in collective action for community betterment: in a word it is entrepreneurial*' (1998, p. 490).

Three strategies to develop entrepreneurial social infrastructure

Flora et al. (1997, p. 627) identified three strategies to develop this kind of social infrastructure. First, legitimising alternatives ensures community members' different opinions, aspirations, and ideas about goals and strategies are being fed into discussions around the community concerning particular issues. This involves airing opinions and managing controversy, depersonalising local politics, and focusing simultaneously on concrete goals and the interactional processes used to achieve them. Communities with a strong entrepreneurial social infrastructure will have diverse groups and strong networks linking them together. These networks ensure that different opinions are actively sought, put on the table, and influence decision-making. Such networks incorporate both strong and weak ties. Weak ties (Granovetter 1973) are especially important here, because these are the ones that connect people with views and opinions that are different from their own.

Activity 4.6

Different views in Yellowleaf

Yellowleaf, the community that was described in Case example 4.1, had made links with diverse groups, including the Islamic community. What were the factors in Yellowleaf that enabled this to happen?

The second ESI strategy, *mobilising resources*, involves people investing their own resources to help the community achieve its goals and complete projects and attract external resources such as investment. Resource contributions include volunteering for boards, in-kind support, and providing funds for various activities. Again, both strong and weak ties are necessary. On the one hand, leaders with strong local ties can engage other residents in projects. In contrast, those with weak local ties but strong external ones through, for example, membership of regional advisory boards of funding bodies can use these to access information and resources to benefit the community.

Activity 4.7

Mobilising community resources

Yellowleaf, the community that was described in Case example 4.1, has a community resource in that it has many older people who have a strong tradition of volunteering. However, this resource is being overlooked as the organisations the volunteers are contributing to, such as the hospital auxiliary, disband. Many of the functions at the hospital that have been fulfilled by volunteers over the years are now being undertaken by paid staff.

Think about it

➤ How do you think Yellowleaf might ensure that these volunteers may continue to contribute if they wish to?

The third strategy involves building *networks* focused on particular tasks that encompass a diverse range of people, interests, and views, are highly interconnected internally and with external networks, and are open to new people and ideas. Although such networks are the medium through which trust is developed (Flora 1998, p. 492), most have both positive (inclusive) and negative (exclusionary) consequences. They should include connections to, and between, groups that are marginalised (or 'outsiders') in the community, because these, too, have useful ideas and resources to contribute to the task at hand. Further, such networks should embody norms of reciprocity and cooperativeness.

Social capital

Social capital, the final component of a community's social infrastructure, is the extent to which relations within it are characterised by trust, reciprocity, and cooperativeness (Bourdieu 1985; Coleman 1988; Portes 1998; Putnam 1995).

While social patterning describes how people are linked together (who interacts with whom), social capital refers to the nature of those links (how they interact) (Cheers et al. 2004). This is how one participant in the community strength study saw it:

> And the footy [football] is that family get-together. You don't ... have to keep track of your kids. If you get a kid this big, you will get a kid this big who will want to push your kid in the pusher all day. The only time you see them is when they want money ... you know that your kids are going to be safe because the community is looking after them. (Cheers et al. 2004, p. 151)

Social capital is a positive resource for communities. Much of the writing about it show limited insight. First, it fails to capture social capital as a property of a community as a whole (Flora 1998; Hawe and Shiell 2000, p. 871). Social capital is both a property of an individual's networks and a community-level phenomenon that cannot be determined by simply aggregating the social capital available to each individual in it. At the community level, social capital is a property of relations between the people in the community taken as a whole. It is a norm, or an implicit rule, about how people should treat each other.

Second, the concept is frequently defined quite abstractly, so that it is vague and difficult to apply in practice when working with communities (Minkler and Wallerstein 2005, p. 37). Misunderstanding may occur when the concept is used differently by various researchers, policymakers, managers, and practitioners.

Pierre Bourdieu (1985) provided the first contemporary systematic analysis of social capital (Portes 1998, p. 2). He defined it as 'the aggregate of the actual and potential resources which are linked to possession of a durable network of more or less institutionalised relationships of mutual acquaintance and recognition' (Portes 1998, p. 2, quoting Bourdieu 1985, p. 248).

According to Bourdieu, then, social capital can be understood at both the individual and the group (and community) level. Putnam (1993, p. 35), too, defined social capital as 'features of social organisation, such as networks, norms, and trust that facilitate coordination and cooperation for mutual benefit'. There is general agreement, then, that it is the elements or qualities of the social relationships that infer social capital.

One implication is that various individuals, families, groups, and sub-populations can have different levels of access to it. For example, those in wealthy and powerful families, including the children, usually have greater access to social capital in a community than marginalised and low-income people, and those from ethnic and cultural minority groups.

Much of the writing about social capital regards it as entirely good for people and communities. However, as several researchers have pointed out, high community social capital can have negative consequences for some individuals (Edwards et al. 2003). Here is an example of how it can be difficult for some individuals in a community to benefit from high levels of social capital.

CASE EXAMPLE 4.4

Can everyone benefit from high levels of social capital?

Brenda has experienced serious domestic violence and is still living with it. She has few emotional or financial resources to invest in social relationships. While she has been invited to join several community organisations, she has no transport, and has little energy, time, money, or capacity to invest in the social relationships that would give her access to the community's social capital. In other words, while there may well be networks in the community with high levels of trust, solidarity, and norms that support reciprocity, she may feel and be excluded because of her inability to reciprocate.

In the public health literature, there has been a proliferation of articles that apply the concept social capital to, and assess its utility for, population health research (Moore et al. 2005, p. 1330). For instance, some research suggests that social capital at the community level may be a mechanism through which income levels affect health status (Kawachi et al. 1997). Nevertheless, Moore et al. (2005, p. 1331) suggest that there is insufficient debate and analysis of how public health research has used the concept, that discussion is dominated by only a few articles, and that alternative, potentially more useful, ways of conceptualising social capital, such as Coleman's (1988) use of rational-choice theory, have not been considered. Moore et al. (2005, p. 1332) go on to argue that it is this lack of critical analysis that has resulted in disenchantment with the concept in public health. For instance, research concerning social capital as a predictor of health status invariably measures social capital at a population level, which means aggregating individual perceptions and characteristics. This tends to produce unconvincing associations. Consequently, detailed understanding of which particular community- and group-level variables comprise or conduce to social capital has not been forthcoming.

Yet, despite the difficulties involved in understanding and measuring the concept, social capital is useful for describing the non-material social capacities of communities that we know are so important in various development projects. It also has practical value to local people doing concrete health and human services projects, provided that they can identify what it means from their own collective perspective.

Activity 4.8

Yellowleaf's social capital

Yellowleaf's newly arrived residents with refugee status come from diverse cultural backgrounds and are fluent in several languages other than English. A high school is thinking of introducing a broader choice of languages, but is concerned that there will not be qualified teachers available.

Think about it

➤ Do you think that Yellowleaf's social capital (its relations characterised by trust, reciprocity, and cooperativeness) could help the high school advance its language program?

Practice tip 4.3

Define social capital with the community you are working with so that everyone understands what it means.

Assessing community capacity

Before we can assess or build community capacity, we have to understand it. The community strength framework underpins our understanding of community capacity. As discussed earlier in this chapter, we can distinguish between the community resources a community has that can potentially be used for development, and the community's ability to use them for these purposes in changing economic, social, and environmental contexts (Cheers, Cock, Hylton Keele et al. 2005).

Community capacity is defined as '[T]he resources a community has that potentially can be used for a specified purpose, and the community's ability to use these for this purpose in changing economic, social, and environmental contexts' (Cheers, Kruger and Trigg, 2005, p. 14). Community resources include, for example, financial assets, physical infrastructure (facilities and equipment), individual knowledge and skills, relations among people and organisations, access to services, and community attitudes.

The distinction that we have made between community resources and capabilities has also been made in public health, although with different terminology. For instance, Goodman et al. (1998, p. 260) distinguished between capacity for health development as a potential state (resources) and competence as an active state (capabilities). Capacity, they suggested, is similar to community readiness, which if skilfully developed (competence) generates action.

In sum, then, community capacity comprises all the factors that support a community taking action on a development issue, such as implementing a new health or community service program. It is the composite of community resources and community capabilities.

Frameworks and measures

Several frameworks have been developed to measure and profile community capacity. Most of these are specific to particular social fields, or sectors, such as health promotion (Labonte and Laverack 2001) and natural resource management (Smith et al. 2005). Both quantitative and qualitative profiles of community capacity have a place. With quantitative measures, we can analyse how various capacities are associated with other quantitative measures such as health status, economic growth, service levels, and service access. They also provide an opportunity to precisely measure changes in capacity over time, devise interventions to increase it, and assess outcomes of these interventions.

Qualitative measures, on the other hand, help us to understand the complex interrelationships among various community capacities, and provide detailed information for strategic planning (Bush et al. 2002, p. 9). Some frameworks include both quantitative and qualitative measures. Chapter 6 provides further information about five approaches for community capacity-building including the Asset Based Community Development framework (Kretzmann and McKnight 1993).

Assessing community capacity for health promotion

Goodman et al. (1998) identified dimensions of community capacity in order to assess capacity in relation to health promotion. Their Community Life Framework (http://www.community-life.org.au/docs/capacity_building.pdf) includes the following community capacities: participation and leadership; skills, resources; social and interagency networks; sense of community, understanding community history; community power; community values; and critical reflection.

Labonte and Laverack (2001 p. 116) also developed a framework and an instrument after reviewing theoretical and empirical models of community capacity for health promotion, including Goodman et al. (1998), and a community action research project involving community members, expert opinion, and health practitioners' views. They identified nine capacity domains: participation; leadership; organisational structures; problem assessment; resource mobilisation; asking why problems occurred; links with others; role of outside agents; and program management.

For their Community Capacity Index (CCI), Bush et al. (2002, p. 4) defined community capacity as 'a collection of characteristics and resources which, when combined, improve the ability of a community to recognise, evaluate and address key problems'. They grouped capacities into four domains: network partnerships; knowledge transfer; problem solving; and infrastructure. The Index measures levels and indicators of capacity within each of these domains.

McLean et al. (2001) measured community capacity to effectively plan, implement, and evaluate health-promotion activities through surveys of individuals and organisations. The surveys provided some indication of the level of practitioners' and organisational leaders' knowledge and skill with regard to health promotion, but they did not conceptualise other capacities, such as resources, attitudes, and values. A later development was a 'health promotion practitioner capacity checklist' to assist health practitioners to determine their level of understanding of their tasks.

It is important to distinguish between instruments that attempt to measure all of a community's social capacities and those that focus on particular ones such as community leadership. The latter are very useful for understanding and measuring specific components of working with communities, such as developing effective partnerships with local opinion leaders, but are less useful for gaining a more comprehensive understanding of community-level capacities such as values, attitudes, community narratives, and how these support or work against development. Other approaches start with a generic concept of community

Practice tip 4.4

Choose an assessment template from the many available that you and the community are comfortable with and is relevant to the specific task. There is no one way to assess community capacity.

capacity, and develop instruments to measure all capacities at the community level. One of these is the Community Capacity Assessment Template of the Department of Primary Industries and Resources South Australia (PIRSA).

Community Capacity Assessment Template

This template starts from the assumption that people need a reliable profile of their communinity's existing capacity in order to plan to strengthen it, and builds on earlier conceptual and applied work (Black and Hughes 2001; McKnight and Kretzmann 2005).

The electronically based community capacity audit/assessment template (Cheers, Cock, Hylton Keele et al. 2005)[1] was developed initially to profile capacity to support local primary industries; however, the broader-based assessment template latest version (C 2007)[2] has a broader community base for measuring a community's capacities, and can be used to support a number of purposes including maintenance of effective health and social services.

With the assistance of a trained facilitator, self-selected community members (the Assessment Group) use the template to measure seventeen capacities in each of eight social fields. The process of conducting the assessment is important, and PIRSA provides guidelines on how this should be done. Consistently with community interaction theory, introduced in Chapter 2, on which the template is based, community members collectively assess capacity. By contrast, viewing community as simply the aggregation of individuals and organisations would motivate an individually focused survey-based approach to measuring capacity.

The template is designed to measure and profile community capacity for each sector and for the community as a whole. The term 'sector' is common in health and human services planning, and is defined for the template as a sphere of human activity in a community. In the language of community interaction theory, a sector is a social field.

The eight fields

Fields identified for the template are:

1 social organisation (community field);
2 health and human services;
3 education;
4 natural resources;
5 business;
6 primary industry;
7 arts and entertainment; and
8 sport and recreation.

This is only one example of how sectors may be defined. In other communities of place and of interest, and for assessments conducted for other purposes, community sectors may be identified quite differently.

The seventeen capacities

The template identifies seventeen capacities, each of which is described below:

1   Mass is the number and range of services and organisations in the sector.
2   Programs are the projects or activities run by the sector.
3   Access is how easily people can participate in sector activities or events.
4   Information is how a community finds out about activities and services.
5   Marketing is about attracting people to the organisations and services in the sector.
6   Resources are financial, human, physical, and in-kind assets available to the sector.
7   Facilities are the permanent infrastructure required to provide services, run organisations and use equipment.
8   Equipment is the hardware used in social interaction.
9   Management is governance issues, processes, and organisational skills.
10 Leadership is the ability of an individual to influence, motivate, and enable others to contribute toward the effectiveness and success of the organisations/sector/community.
11 Networks and relationships are the inter-linkages and interpersonal relationships that people build and benefit from by exchanging information and ideas.
12 Government is the support from local, state, and the Australian Government, and includes community plans, policy formation and administration.
13 Social capital is mutual trust, reciprocity, cooperation, and collaboration.
14 Advocacy is the act of representing an issue, idea or person, and includes representing the interests and needs of the sector.
15 Inclusiveness is mediating, harnessing, and embracing different views and opinions for integrated and collective action.
16 Ethics are theological or moral viewpoints, and include principles, values, and beliefs based on what people consider to be right or wrong.
17 Community spirit is about having pride in the sector, and includes caring, welcoming, and friendliness.

For each capacity, the template measures:

➤   its *strength*, using indicators provided on the template (CS in Figure 4.2);
➤   its *importance* to total community capacity (CI in Figure 4.2); and
➤   its *contribution* (CC in Figure 4.2) to total community capacity (a composite of strength and importance).

FIGURE 4.2   Yellowleaf's community capacities for the health and human services sector

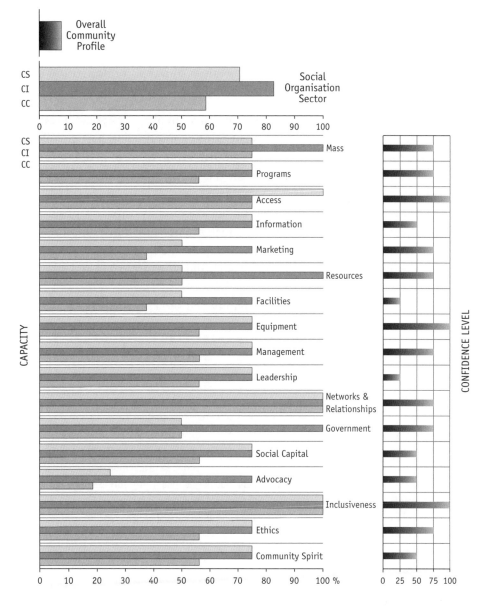

As a validity check, it also measures how confident the assessors are in their assessment of each capacity. Various capacity profiles are generated. For capacity building, the most useful are:

1   the total capacity of each sector;
2   each capacity for the entire community;
3   the capacities in each sector; and
4   each capacity across sectors.

Figure 4.2 presents the profile of capacities for the health and human services sector in Yellowleaf.[3]

Using the Community Capacity Assessment Template

Communities use the template to collect, analyse, and report information as part of a cyclical, six-step community capacity-building process:

1 Preparing to conduct the assessment; this involves selecting a qualified facilitator, assembling the Assessment Group, and briefing participants. The assessment is conducted by a representative group of local people assembled by the community according to specified criteria.
2 Conducting the assessment in a workshop.
3 Analysing assessment data, constructing community capacity profiles, and reporting results to the community, which are done by the facilitator.
4 Conducting a planning workshop involving the facilitator, Assessment Group, and other community members in which profiles are presented and a capacity-building plan is formulated.
5 Implementing the plan by the community and service providers.
6 Periodic monitoring of progress through further assessments.

Notes

1   The template was developed by the *Department of Primary Industries and Resources South Australia (PIRSA)*, which commissioned *Rural Solutions SA* and the *Centre for Rural Health and Community Development* at the University of South Australia to undertake some of the work. *The Government of SA* holds the copyright for the general template and all derivatives of the original that use any of the original ideas, theories, or layouts. Reproduction of any part of PIRSA's community capacity assessment process, including the template, can only be done with written permission from PIRSA.

2   In 2007, the template was broadened to include seventeen capacities. The *Government of SA* holds the copyright for the template version C 2007.

3   A fictional town discussed in Case example 4.1.

SUMMARY

This chapter has introduced the concept 'community capacity' as the resources that are inherent in the community and the community's capability to use them. There are three aspects of this definition. First, we have distinguished between community resources and capabilities. Second, we have included resources both internal and external to the community, provided that the community can access them. Third, we have distinguished community resources and individual and organisational resources. Community resources are 'out there' for community members generally to use, rather than being available only to those in particular families, groups, organisations, or businesses. Several concepts related to community capacity were also introduced—community strength, entrepreneurial social infrastructure, social patterning, and social capital—and some of the challenges in applying them to actual health and social care projects were identified.

We identified several frameworks and instruments devised to profile and measure community capacity specifically in health. Then we presented in some detail a particular electronic template to measure community capacity as a generic, whole-of-community construct. People in a community use this template to assess, through a workshop process, the strength of particular capacities in particular sectors, their importance to particular tasks, how confident they are about their assessments, and the contribution that each capacity makes to total community capacity.

USEFUL WEBSITES

Assessing and building community capacity

Community builders' resource exchange: http://www.commbuild.org/

Community capacity section of the Life Framework: http://www.community-life.org.au

The United Nations Development Programme downloadable booklet on Capacity Assessment: http://mirror.undp.org/magnet/cdrb/

The Community Development Exchange: (http://www.community-life.org.au/docs/capacity_building.pdf)

Department for Victorian Communities—Community-building resources: http://www.communitybuilding.vic.gov.au/index.shtml

NSW Government community builders: http://www.communitybuilders.nsw.gov.au/

Community capacity for health development

The Australian Department of Health and Ageing's Building Healthy Communities is a guide for people in small communities who want to try new ways to make a difference to chronic disease at a local level: http://www.health.gov.au/internet/wcms/publishing.nsf/Content/ruralhealth-pubs-BHC.htm

PART 2

Approaches to Working with Communities

Part 1 presented the key principles of working with communities and the theoretical framework to understand the aspects of community functioning that are relevant to community health and social care development. The focus was on the community: its social structures, including patterns of networking, power structures, and capacities and resources to undertake development.

In Part 2, the focus is on the approaches and frameworks used to work with communities in developing community health and social wellbeing. Chapter 5 constructs a typology to define, illustrate, and clarify the different conceptual approaches. Chapter 6 presents five practice frameworks from community development, health promotion, and rural development practice to illustrate the steps involved in practice. Chapter 7 demonstrates two government approaches to working with communities: community services development (CSD) and community engagement. While the focus in Chapter 7 is on community and health service and program development, community engagement is practised in education, natural resource management, the arts, and in all types of social and land-use planning.

CHAPTER 5

Conceptual Approaches to Working with Communities

Introduction

This chapter will present four conceptual approaches to working with communities:

➤ the contributions approach;
➤ the instrumental approach;
➤ the community empowerment approach; and
➤ the developmental approach.

Four conceptual approaches

This chapter presents a typology of four conceptual approaches to working with communities that are apparent in community health and social care development. Each differs quite considerably with regard to leadership, the respective roles for communities, governments, practitioners, and the decision-making processes, and each may be effective given the policy context, the task to be achieved, and the community.

In Chapter 1, we presented a definition of community health and social care development as 'communities working together with practitioners and governments in assessing social and health needs and issues, and organising and implementing effective strategies to meet those needs' (Zakus and Lysack 1998, p. 2). While we would all agree that this is what community health and social care development is, the definition brings us no closer to understanding the diverse thinking about how best to achieve this.

Most often, this thinking is not made explicit, and the rhetoric about working with communities in policy documents implies, rather than defines, what approach is to be taken. Can 'working with communities' be seen as implementing an evidence-based intervention with a group of older adults to help prevent accidental falls? Or is it to be seen as a process of community change, one in which groups of local residents will devise solutions to address health and wellbeing issues, and get involved in implementing services and programs? Or is it both of these things?

Uncovering the implicit expectations about who should lead the initiatives and how community residents are to be involved helps reveal the underlying approach. Clarity about the approach assists in understanding whether the approach is appropriate, given the desired outcome in the particular context. A mismatch between the conceptual approach and the desired outcome is one of the reasons some processes in working with communities are ineffective.

In practice, the approaches are not discrete, and elements of each approach may and should coexist. It is never an 'either-or' situation. It is a matter of choosing the approach that is feasible and appropriate, given the policy environment, the community concerned—whether it is a community of place or of interest—and

TABLE 5.1   Four conceptual approaches to working with communities

The contributions approach	The contributions approach considers participation as voluntary contributions to a project, rather than decision-making about the project. Professional developers, usually external to the community concerned, lead participation. (Oakley and Marsden 1984; Oakley 1989).
The instrumental approach	The instrumental approach defines health and wellbeing as an end result rather than as a process. The end result is effective strategies that improve health and wellbeing for consumers. Consumer and community involvement are interventions designed to achieve outcomes for communities in the most equitable and effective manner. Participation is usually led by professionals. (Rifkin 1986, 1996).
The community empowerment approach	The community empowerment approach seeks to empower and support communities, individuals, and groups to take greater control over issues that affect their health and wellbeing. It includes the notions of personal development, consciousness-raising and social action. (Williams and Labonte 2003).
The developmental approach	The developmental approach conceptualises health and social care development as an interactive, evolutionary process, embedded in a community, in which local people have an active role. Through their involvement, tasks that they consider important are achieved. The developmental approach is underpinned by principles of social justice. (Cheers and Luloff 2001; Ife and Tesoriero 2006).

the outcomes that the key stakeholders wish to achieve. If it is not obvious how community members are to be involved in an initiative, and whether or not they should be at all, or how far communities can 'have a say', then the underlying conceptual approach is not clear and it is very unlikely that the community can be effectively involved.

Information about these conceptual approaches has been drawn from a wide range of sources including primary health care (Legge et al. 1996), community building for health (Minkler 2005), health promotion (Labonte 1994), social development (Midgley 1986a), rural development (Krishna et al. 1997), and community development (Cheers and Luloff 2001; Ife and Tesoriero 2006). Table 5.1 clarifies these conceptual approaches.

Practice tip 5.1

Make sure you find out before you begin working with a community how far the community can have a say in the program directions.

The contributions approach

The distinguishing feature of the contributions approach is that it involves voluntary donations of time and expertise, for example, labour, local knowledge and skills, access to local networks, money, and other in-kind contributions from local residents. However, there is usually no expectation that contributors will be influential in decision-making about how the resources are used, or in the project directions. For example, community fund-raising is a strategy for purchasing medical equipment for a hospital. Although the funds are essential, the decisions about what equipment to purchase are made without community involvement (Short 1989). Case example 5.1, used to demonstrate the contributions approach, is about the early years of the Sera's Women's Shelter in Townsville, North Queensland.

Oakley and Marsden (1984, pp. 17–19), in reviewing interpretations of participation in rural development in developing countries, identified the contributions approach to community participation as a dominant paradigm. Material contributions and voluntary labour from rural communities were often fundamental to a project getting off the ground, but participation in making decisions about the project rarely occurred. Development personnel continued to be influential in how the contributions were used, and local people were not expected to take part in shaping the program or criticising its content (Oakley and Marsden 1984, p. 19, citing Economic Commission for Latin America 1973).

CASE EXAMPLE 5.1

Sera's Women's Shelter

Sera's Women's Shelter has always been a service that provides accommodation and support for women with or without children who are leaving a violent or otherwise intolerable domestic situation. Sera's Shelter commenced in 1975 and was part of a significant movement that exposed the serious problem of domestic violence and sexual abuse. Recognising the need for a safe, secure, and emotionally supportive environment for women and their children in North Queensland, the Women's Electoral Lobby, a local government social worker, and other women worked to set up a shelter. The group rented a house, staffed it with volunteers and, for the first few months, ran the Shelter on privately donated funds.

While the momentum to keep the service going was strong, the obstacles were significant. Funding became a serious issue, and in the late 1970s an operational grant from government was obtained. However, the grant came with strings attached in that to access the grant the Shelter needed to provide 12.5 per cent of the funds itself. This represented $200 per week, which took a large amount of the workers' time and affected their most important role, working with the women. Each week, Shelter workers and volunteers could be seen selling raffle tickets outside the local supermarket. In addition, the shelter continued to rely on donations of money, expertise, clothing, household linen and generous support of the overnight volunteers.

Today, Sera's Shelter has reasonably secure ongoing funding. While it provides a comprehensive and responsive service, community contributions remain an important aspect. (Sera's Women's Shelter 2005)

Think about it

➤ How does this case example demonstrate a contributions approach to service development?

➤ What are the advantages and disadvantages of accepting government funding?

➤ Should the service continue to include community contributions?

➤ There are now no overnight volunteers at Sera's and some of them miss the opportunity to contribute. What is your view about using volunteers at this service?

Practice tip 5.2

Sometimes community contributions are important because they encourage a sense of ownership of the service and help people to feel connected. But this must be balanced with adequate resources to provide an effective service.

The contributions approach to development evolved for pragmatic rather than ideological reasons. In the context of scarce resources to deal with serious social, health, and economic problems, local communities could be seen by governments to generate extra resources. Midgley (1986b, p. 40) describes this as the manipulative mode of social development, used in order to reduce the project costs to the state.

In an era in which governments are seeking to reduce expenditure on human and health services, instances of the contributions approach in both health and social

CASE EXAMPLE 5.2

A contributions approach to community health development

Source: Zakus 1998, pp. 481–92

In a resource-poor rural area of Mexico, the Health Ministry was challenged to extend primary health care, and so used local people to set up local health posts and run health care groups on a voluntary basis. However, the support provided was minimal and training and resources were inadequate. Local people were not involved in setting targets, and therefore the outcomes were limited. Community involvement was a strategy implemented entirely for its utility in supplying resources that the Ministry lacked, rather than for any intrinsic or democratic values.

Think about it

➤ How can this example be seen as a contributions approach to health development?

➤ What do you see as the problems in maintaining the community contributions?

care development are continuing. Even when communities are the driving force behind a project, government may perceive that if the community wants the service, then it is their role is to contribute. Community-based programs and volunteer input can be seen as 'services on the cheap' (Ife and Tesoriero 2006, p. 13).

In some country areas in Australia, there is a long history of communities contributing financially and through in-kind resources to their health services, notably hospitals, without necessarily being involved in broader decision-making about them. Collins (2001) writes of the notion of 'voluntarism' in country Victoria, where, in the 1990s, the State government sought the assistance of rural communities to implement changes to the health system. This appeared to mean that if the communities wished to retain the same level of service, they must be increasingly willing to fund these themselves. This approach involved devolution of what was originally government responsibly for funding to rural communities.

Another example is the increasing level of community involvement in maintaining general practice services in country towns in Australia, where there are serious general practitioner recruitment issues (Wilkinson 2000). In order to attract doctors to rural towns, some communities, through their local hospital boards and other organisations, may contribute their time, financial resources, housing assistance, and practice infrastructure. There is an acknowledgment that if the town cannot retain a general practitioner, then this will negatively affect the future of the local hospital. The hospital is often a major employer in the town and contributes to long-term economic and social sustainability. A research participant explains this issue:

> The general practice is important, just grist to the mill. Every little thing you lose in a town is important. Survival is about a feeling of confidence rather than economics sometimes. If a doctor comes here then that is something positive; if that goes everybody gets all depressed and thinks it will be the school next. Actually it is not all that different for me to drive to go to the doctor but you feel good about going to the doctor in your local town. For some people it is really an important thing, as they can't drive. (Taylor 2004, p. 111)

Reciprocity and mutual benefits from contributions

The contributions approach relies upon some mutual benefit in order for communities to continue to keep contributing. Short (1989) critiqued community participation in a regional area in Australia where $1.5 million dollars was raised to purchase a linear accelerator for the local hospital. The benefit to the community was stressed as the opportunity to access health care in the regional centre rather than travelling to the city. Being able to access human and health services locally is a strong motivator to prompt people to contribute. In these examples, rural communities contribute to supporting their health services because of their desire not only to have access to a range of services, but also because health services contribute significantly to community sustainability.

The notion of reciprocity is evident in most volunteer programs, where there are reciprocal benefits both at the community and the individual level (Creyton et al. 2005). Training for volunteers in leadership, or the specific activities involved, may be a benefit, and volunteers may obtain personal satisfaction from the volunteering experience. At the community level, traditions of civic participation may be reinforced and new organisations and social networks established. People may gain a sense of achievement and community connectedness when activities are successful. However, there are critiques of the contributions approach, particularly where there is there is little reciprocity involved.

Critiques of the contributions approach

The contributions approach is usually criticised on three grounds. First, it is generally inconsistent with a redistribution of power and resources from those devising and implementing the service or program to local residents (Dwyer 1989, p. 60). Communities are seen as 'contributors' rather than active participants in these partnerships. Therefore, it is inconsistent with the maxim that a redistribution of resources is to be one outcome of community participation, especially in the context of the development of third world countries (Midgley 1986b, p. 24).

Second, the contributions approach to community participation may not be sustainable. While communities may wish to maintain their involvement, unless there are positive outcomes and people are able to have a say in how their donations are used, their commitment may diminish. Even if volunteers do want to continue, they may not be able to afford to. For example, lay volunteers working without financial incentives extended a tuberculosis screening program in a resource-limited, high disease-burden setting in South Africa. However, they had to earn an income and could not keep up their voluntary contributions. 'A major hindrance to community participation in developing countries is the desire for remuneration by the lay volunteers. There is evidence to suggest that in the absence of appropriate incentives, attrition rates in lay worker programs tend to be high after the initial novelty wears off' (Kironde and Kahitimbanyi 2002, p. 22).

Third, community participation can be a 'double-edged sword'. People may be called on to do things for themselves, deflecting attention from the government resource issues that have brought about the need for this approach (Herbert-Cheshire 2000; Ife and Tesoriero 2006). In talking about some Third World health development, Foster (1982, p. 186) critiques the contributions approach as 'rural development on the cheap', and Morgan (2001, pp. 221) refers to the 'utilitarian' efforts of aid organisations or governments to use community resources to offset the costs of providing services. Stone (1992, p. 412) adds to this sentiment: 'The rhetoric of community participation can be used as a substitute for government responsibility in public health, or as a mask that shields national and international inequalities of wealth and power, which are the real causes of poverty and ill-health in the third world.'

The instrumental approach

The second conceptual approach—the instrumental approach—is the dominant approach to community health and social care development in Australia currently. This is driven by the need to provide health and human services within a market model of service provision (Taylor 1999). The market model is described by Kettner and Martin (1986, pp. 35–6) as

> a set of policies and practices that encourages competition among potential contractors; and, where like contractors are competing to provide a like service, price is the determining factor. The market model places a high value on cost efficiency. An agency following the market model would emphasise the development of criteria for measuring efficiency and effectiveness and negotiate with a high degree of specificity on issues of performance expectations, program design, budget and cost.

In order to achieve efficiencies in health and human service provision, extensive economic reforms and public sector restructuring has occurred in Australia and internationally. Public services have been privatised, contractual arrangements now separate purchasers of services and providers, and there has been the introduction of competition to allocate resources (Hancock 1999). The rise of managerialism in health and human services, with its emphasis on managers achieving strategic outputs with tight control over budgets, is a related development. Policy analysts agree that financing is the major driving force behind these reforms (Mahnken 2001). In this environment, the dominant approach to working with communities is one where the emphasis is on meeting clearly defined targets or outcomes from community participation rather than establishing mutually beneficial participatory processes that may extend beyond the primary objective.

In instrumental approaches, 'working with communities' is conceptualised as 'community' or 'consumer' participation—involvement by individuals, groups, and communities according to a strategy designed by professionals to improve health or social wellbeing. The achievement of a predetermined goal or target is seen as more important than the act of participation. Participation becomes a means to an end, and the 'end' is meeting of an objective that has already been defined in strategic planning exercises or in policy.

Strategies for participation may be designed to effectively target services, or to achieve greater clarity around unmet needs, or to engage volunteers in program delivery. In this approach, working with communities is an intervention, with the 'intervention' being conceptualised into some kind of planning process, or program implementation, with the accompanying paraphernalia of objectives, budgets, and control. Oakley (1989, p. 10) describes this approach:

> The results of the participation in the shape of the predetermined targets are more important than the act of participation. Government and development agencies responsible for providing services and with the power to control resources see participation as a means of improving the efficiency of their service delivery systems, which will benefit both the provider and consumer.

A distinguishing feature of the approach is that it is undertaken using methods consistent with a professional power-base, and processes are activated and directed by professionals. Rifkin (1986, p. 241) described three approaches to working with communities as the 'medical', 'health services', and 'community development' approaches. More lately, Rifkin (1996, p. 80) distinguished between approaches that are target-oriented (the medical and health services approach), and those that are intended to empower local people to gain resources and, eventually, control over their own lives (the community development approach). The targeted approach—a top-down approach to working with communities—is consistent with contributions and instrumental approaches.

> The [target-oriented] approach is one in which planners/professionals decide the specific objectives of a health program and then attempt to convince community people to actively accept these objectives. Two distinct variations can be described. In the first professionals try to convince community people to accept a specific health intervention. The second variation is the situation in which planners/health professionals want a community contribution to the program they have defined. Both variations expect local people to participate, within the context defined by the planners/professionals to bring about improvement in their health status. (Rifkin 1996, pp. 80–1)

Top-down programs follow a predetermined cycle, commencing with the overall design of the project or service, objective setting, selection of an appropriate strategy, implementation and management, and program evaluation. Strategic plans involve a linear approach, moving from overall aims to objectives, and then to activities. This simplifies the complexity of the planning process and meets requirements for clearly defined outcomes. While there is always the possibility of some adaptation at the local level, this approach inevitably produces tension between the goals of strategic plans and the needs and priorities of communities. This 'top-down–bottom-up' tension is endemic to the instrumental approach to working with communities. Case example 5.3 illustrates this tension.

CASE EXAMPLE 5.3

The Health and Social Welfare councils of SA

Source: Baum et al. 1997

In the late 1980s, Health and Social Welfare councils were established in South Australia, aiming to enable community input into health planning and promotion. The government health department provided a secretariat and a part-time project worker for each council. Increasingly, councils became focused on providing input into health planning at every level of government, and it became difficult to maintain a community-initiated agenda. Members felt they were 'owned' by government, and it was the goals of health administrators that were in focus, with little space to meet the needs of community members.

Think about it

➤ How does this case example demonstrate an instrumental approach to participation?
➤ Why did members see difficulties in raising community issues?
➤ What problems might arise in the future with these councils if the agenda is only focused to government needs?

Practice tip 5.3

Balancing a community and a government or organisational agenda is always a challenge, and there must be compromises.

Critiques of the approach

Fundamentally, critiques of the instrumental approach to working with communities are related to the current context of health and human services delivery, which demands this approach. One ongoing problem is that communities feel that consultation about needs and priorities is becoming increasingly 'token' (Quartermaine 2003). Often there is a brief information session during which community members are informed about a new program, but rarely is there involvement in decision-making at a stage where community input can have an impact.

It is acknowledged that genuinely asking people for their opinions about important issues and reaching consensus within the tight timeframes imposed by strategic planning deadlines is difficult. It is even more difficult to have the community input inform policy. Goals and objectives may well have already been determined, and community input may be interpreted as consultation to seek commitment to those goals and objectives (Baum 1996; Johnson 1996).

New programs designed by governments to improve community health inevitably involve predetermined indicators against which program success will be measured. Meeting these indicators necessitates a focus on a particular type of intervention, and a particular health issue. The move to fund tightly targeted initiatives at the community level is critiqued in that it necessitates a level of specificity that is difficult for many communities to meet. Often those communities who are most at need of the intervention are unable to access funding.

What is meant by community in an instrumental approach?

This book has provided a definition of community in Chapter 2 that is useful in undertaking community health and social care development. However, the operationalisation of 'community' in the instrumental approach is problematic. It can be anything—populations, organisations, or groups of consumers, patients, or clients. This makes it very difficult to embed practice in working with communities in a theoretical framework such as community interaction theory.

Generally, in health and human service policy, it is the involvement of consumers in planning and program development rather than communities that is sought (Taylor et al. 2006a, p. 38). In the World Health Organisation Declaration of Alma Ata, it was communities that were in focus; communities were to be supported to identify their health needs and work in partnership to address them (WHO 1978). Since this Declaration, there has been a shift from 'community' to 'consumer', and this is consistent with a managerialist approach to service delivery.

Many professionals find the concept of 'community' difficult to unpack because of the current emphasis on health and social care as a transaction between themselves as providers and individual clients as consumers of a product. They are not trained to 'think community' either, and don't have the conceptual tools to do so. Therefore, the relationship with a patient or client is defined as a one-on-one engagement, and may imply dependence between recipients of services and the providing agencies. A 'consumer' is an individualised concept, emphasising the notion of health and social care as a product rather than a process, and a consumer as an individual who uses the product (Ryan, 2001, p. 105). These constructions inevitably place an emphasis on individual responsibility for health and social wellbeing. This, in turn, results in an interpretation of health and social problems, and their solutions in individual terms, and there is no collective or 'community' implied.

A top-down approach

Another criticism of the instrumental approach is that it generally does not result in a transfer of power from professionals to communities (Rifkin 1996). There is no doubt that the current approach to health development and primary health care is top-down, with health professionals controlling the method and process of community participation. Structures used to obtain community input are often dominated by professionals or policymakers who lead the agenda, which is designed to meet their needs. Establishing structures such as advisory councils and the like is seen as a means to meet the official discourse of participation without actually having to embark on administrative reform that would be necessary if communities were to have real input.

In the United Kingdom, Milewa et al. (1999) found that although structures had been established to gain citizens' views, health administrators still regarded their views about needs and priorities as more relevant. A health administrator in Milewa et al.'s (1999, p. 454) study illustrates this point:

> It isn't our job to be 'champions of the people'—that implies a populist approach … Our job is to make rational decisions based upon evidence about what the best value for money is in terms of directing limited healthcare resources towards the greatest need. And that isn't always going to be popular with the general public.

Practice tip 5.4

Usually it is possible to meet both an organisational agenda and an aspect of a community agenda concurrently, but this requires careful negotiation.

The community empowerment approach

The third conceptual approach is the community empowerment approach. Empowerment literally means the process of giving power or authority to an individual or group (Heller 1989, p. 8). However, the term can be used loosely, and it is very difficult to find an adequate definition of it. In current health promotion practice, 'empowerment' can be used to describe any development process or activity, such as skills training or the development of management techniques, which might have some impact upon people's ability to deal with different political and administrative systems (Kahssay and Oakley 1999, p. 7). The result of this is that it may become a 'catch-all' phrase that means whatever someone wants it to mean (Yeo 1993, p. 226, citing O'Neil 1989).

Rifkin (1996) had a precise understanding of community empowerment in health promotion and planning. She considered that empowerment of community participants involved health professionals giving up their dominant position in programs, equivalent to power shifting from professionals to non-professionals or lay people.

> Basically, the empowerment frame of reference sees community participation as the result of community people, essentially the poor, gaining information, access to resources and eventually control over their own lives rather than being dominated by the authorities (elites) by whom they have been exploited. (Rifkin 1996, p. 82)

An excellent review of the use of the term 'empowerment' in health promotion and health planning, and its relationship to people's participation, occurs in a literature review by Rifkin, Lewando-Hundt and Draper (2000). In summary, these authors demonstrate the alignment of the concept of empowerment, in its broadest sense, with a bottom-up approach to community participation in development. Local people become involved in a process of determining priorities and solving problems, and, in the process, increase their knowledge and skill base in addition to achieving a sense of control over their environment. There is an emphasis on the process of participation as a process of change, as well as an outcome in terms of task achievement.

Empowerment is a central construct for health promotion (Bracht 1999; Labonte 1994; Laverack and Labonte 2000; Williams and Labonte 2003), with conceptual underpinning coming from the Ottawa Charter for Health Promotion (WHO 1986), Alinsky (1969), and Freire (1996). The Ottawa Charter identified the fundamental conditions and resources for community health, and identified five principles, one of which was to empower communities to be able to make local decisions (McMurray 1999, p. 16–17). Current interpretations of empowerment within health promotion include the notions of personal development, consciousness-raising, and social action, which are necessary if individuals and communities are to be able to influence the issues that affect their health (Williams and Labonte 2003).

Laverack and Labonte (2000) have developed a framework for health promotion that attempts to meld bottom-up approaches with the top-down approach that characterise current funding programs. The framework is intended to assist health promoters to systematically accommodate community empowerment goals in

CASE EXAMPLE 5.4

Health promotion camps

Source: Pika Wiya Health Service Inc 2004

An Aboriginal Health Service provided a wide range of programs for Aboriginal people from different cultural and linguistic groups in the region to prevent the onset of chronic illness, and help people affected manage their condition. Information about chronic illness self-management was provided at local events and through giving talks at the local schools. Another approach was to consult with community members about their needs and provide information that was directly related to their requests. The organisation found that people were interested in doing this through going away together and having time to talk about issues in a relaxed setting.

Several camps were held where people could discuss health issues obtain relevant information. In this relaxed atmosphere, relationships were built up and people were able to raise more complex problems including poverty, unemployment, and housing. People began to be able to speak of their concerns, especially those about other family members. The relationships between community members and the health professionals who attended the camps became stronger. In learning more about diabetes, one older person reflected, 'If only I knew then what I know now.'

Think about it

➤ How does this case example illustrate an empowerment approach to health promotion?
➤ What might be some of the benefits of this approach?
➤ Why might be some benefits of stronger relationships between health professionals and community members?

program design, objective-setting, strategy selection, strategy implementation and management, and program evaluation. Frameworks developed by Bracht et al. (1999) and Walter (2005) for engaging communities in health-promotion activities, are also based on empowerment principles. Case example 5.4 is an example of a health-promotion program based on principles of empowerment.

Critiques of the approach

It is difficult to find case studies that illustrate changing the nature of power relationships between professionals and marginalised groups. The World Health Organisation, which originally used the term 'empowerment' as involving a redistribution of power from health professionals to local people (WHO 1991, p. 25), later conceptualised community empowerment differently, more as the creation of 'mechanisms for partnerships and the allocation of adequate resources to support those partnerships' (WHO 2000 p. ix). This is quite a move from the challenging statement to health professionals that community involvement in health is limited because of professional control over health information and decision-making.

Cleaver (2001) considers that the term 'empowerment' is used erroneously in development projects as it no longer refers to local residents achieving real power over decision-making.

> The predominant discourses of development now are practical and technical, concerned with project-dictated imperatives of efficiency, rather than empowering. The radical challenging and transformatory edge to empowerment that was originally conceived has been lost, and the concept of action has become individualised, and empowerment depoliticised. (Cleaver 2001, p. 37)

Labonte (2005, p. 85) makes the point that in working to 'empower' a community, we may actually be empowering one community group at the expense of others. For example, empowering a community development association to get more involved in community health planning may alienate community health staff and others who are already centrally involved and regard this as their territory. In working with communities, we tend to work initially with locally powerful people because these people have the resources and influence to coordinate the broad

Practice tip 5.5

Make sure you can explain what you mean by 'empowerment' to those with whom you are working.

community input that is required in developing programs. We may increase the resources of this group at the expense of the disempowered, including those people who use the programs and services that we are developing (Cheers 1998, p. 150).

The developmental approach

A developmental approach to working with communities is one in which local people, usually through collective community-based processes, are actively involved in a project over which they can exert some influence (Oakley and Marsden 1984, p. 19). Participation processes themselves are beneficial both at an individual and community level as participants may gain new skills and build new relationships, thereby increasing community capacity to solve problems together. It is an opportunity for communities to express community agency. Community agency is the sum of purposive acts expressing the capacity of residents to work together for the wellbeing of the entire community (Cheers and Luloff 2001, p. 135): 'Community development focuses on enhancing the quality of life of the whole community—socially, economically, culturally, spiritually and ecologically—by increasing community agency, primarily through broadly based local participation.'

Rifkin (1996 p. 83) refers to the developmental approach as 'bottom up', where participative processes are conceived of as an 'end in itself enabling local people, through involvement and experience, to gain access and control of health care resources'. The key elements of the developmental approach are that local people are involved in decision-making, both the processes of participation and task achievement are valued, and participation results in meeting local participants' objectives.

The developmental approach to participation is apparent in the community development literature (Cheers and Luloff 2001; Ife and Tesoriero 2006, Martinez-Brawley 2000) and rural development literature (Kothari, 1999; Krishna et al. 1997), as well as in Aboriginal and Torres Strait Islander health development (Atkinson 2001; Commonwealth of Australia 2001).

Community development typifies a participatory approach based on social justice principles, which generates and influences policies, planning, and services, and builds residents' personal and collective capacities, and enhances community cohesion (Cheers 1995, p. 3). Cheers defined the principles that underpin community involvement in the development of human services as:

➤ the pursuit of social justice;
➤ the belief that people should control their own destinies as communities, groups, and individuals;

➤ collective action, or the intrinsic importance of people working together to address common problems and issues;

➤ open, democratic decision-making, and

➤ partnership, defined as residents and relevant communities of interest and governments being involved in the development management and provision of services.

The following case example illustrates the key principles of a developmental approach to working with communities—in this case a neighbourhood in a regional city.

CASE EXAMPLE 5.5

Neighbourhood development

Source: Community and Cultural Services Consultancy Unit, Townsville City Council 2001

A neighbourhood in a regional city had a long tradition of involvement in local organisations and networks. It was a community where people knew each other and relationships were strengthened through participation in the local churches, the football club, and meeting informally at each other's houses. Aboriginal and Torres Strait Islander families were involved in many community activities, and all families supported one another. There was employment for most families and little disparity between the living situations of individual families.

There was also a tradition of advocacy about issues affecting the neighbourhood, with the Progress Association taking issues to local and state governments. For example, the association was involved in a campaign to oppose the eviction of public tenants from temporary accommodation. There was evidence of a tight-knit community that had stood together to solve problems.

The opportunity for the neighbourhood to work in partnership with local government was made possible through an urban renewal funding program that had a strong community development approach. Participation occurred very early in the planning for the project through community reference groups for public tenants, homeowners, businesses, and community organisations. Although it was resource-intensive and would need to continue over a long period, local government and other stakeholders all committed to it.

In order to identify the strengths of the community, interviews were held with randomly selected households. Interviewers were from the local school, and were trained and supported in this role. In addition, a survey was distributed to households and businesses in the suburb. A project office was established locally and a newsletter was distributed as a means of communication.

Early in the project, a group of residents met at the school to plan for a neighbourhood centre that would act as a focal point for the community. Support for the group came from many sources including the community development workers at the project office, the primary school, and local government. Now the centre is established, it continues to provide an environment where people can come together to share ideas, skills, knowledge and experience. It also acts to stimulate community involvement in a wide range of issues.

Another aspect of the project was the improvement of recreational facilities and upgrades of open spaces with community involvement in planning and design. Because of the involvement of the community, parks are well used and there are indications of a strong sense of local ownership.

Think about it

➤ How does this case example demonstrate a developmental approach?

➤ Why do you think this approach was chosen by local government?

➤ What are some of the advantages and disadvantages of this approach in this case study?

Examples of a developmental approach are common in Indigenous health. Atkinson (2001) describes a holistic[1] prenatal and perinatal service to young mothers, fathers, and grandmothers provided by a community-controlled Aboriginal and Torres Strait Islander health centre. Clinic group sessions involved health checks for the mothers and babies, and also involved fathers and other children in planning for the families' health, as well as addressing other issues. Transport was provided to and from the clinic, and child care was available. Grandmothers were also involved, and were important guests at a special ceremony where the new baby was welcomed into the community. The program became so popular that it moved to its own accommodation (Atkinson 2001).

Krishna et al. (1997) compiled case studies that demonstrated successful change processes, achieving ongoing social and economic benefits that were locally grounded and involved residents in decision-making. An example is the development of a community-controlled bank in rural Bangladesh. Local people developed banking groups, decided the rules for borrowing and repayment, and monitored repayments. An international development agency supplied a small amount of initial set-up capital, but because of the level of community involvement, the bank became community-owned. The process of acquiring loans led to greater economic independence, as people had been unable to access credit previously. Being involved in a successful banking endeavour enabled local people to gain self-esteem (Yunus 1997, p. 10).

Developmental approaches to community participation in an industrial suburb of Adelaide enabled local people to act together to reduce the level of industrial air and water pollutants, which people considered affected their health. Through a process of community engagement and organisation, a resident action group was formed, which set about to lobby industrial groups in the area. In the longer term, local residents achieved a sense of control over one of the factors that they considered affected their health environment (Tesoriero 1995).

Minkler (2005) and her colleagues write of community organising and community building as a process to facilitate communities to use their voice to define and make their health concerns known and acted upon. The professionals concerned have a critical role to play in helping communities realise their strengths in all aspects of the process of improving health and wellbeing. The community building approach is developmental in that it focuses on a practitioner as part of a community, and using a social justice framework analyses the power structures that contribute to inequities.

Critiques of the approach

Using a developmental approach in working with communities is challenging in an environment that demands the achievement of highly targeted objectives. Government departments face pressures in delivering output performance targets on time. To justify budget requests, government personnel are under pressure to show quick results, especially those that can be quantified. If they choose to adopt a community development approach to some of their service development, then they are relinquishing some degree of control over their ability to deliver their agreed outputs within a specified timeframe. Clearly, the length of time that it takes to encourage participation, to enable people to feel confident enough to participate, and to support a process that may wander at times from the strategic directions required by administrators is an issue. There are rarely sufficient resources to support community involvement, and even if there were, it is very time-consuming to work with marginalised groups to enable them to have a say.

The second problem in using a developmental approach is that the goals and targets that governments require often do not fit with the needs and priorities of the community (Johnson 1996). Practitioners may choose not to consult with the community at all rather than hear about the needs and priorities that cannot be accommodated within government priorities. Governments may be fearful that if communities are to voice their views and take action to meet their perceived needs, then this will result in conflict and competing agendas.

Critiques of the developmental approach argue that advocates for it are primarily ideological and value-oriented rather than pragmatic and performance-oriented (Perlstadt et al. 1998). This view suggests that those who use the developmental approach value the process of building individual and community capacity rather than task accomplishment. Creating an 'either-or' dichotomy results in developmental approaches being seen as time-consuming, impractical, and lacking in strategic focus. Rifkin (1996) suggests that this 'either-or' dichotomy is flawed and that both task achievement and building community capacity can and should coexist.

Note

1   The term 'holistic' is used in Aboriginal health to denote an approach that integrates social, emotional, spiritual and cultural health—it is preferred to the western medical model, which Aboriginal people call the 'body-parts' model.

SUMMARY

This chapter has identified and developed a typology of four conceptual approaches to working with communities. It is important to define these approaches in order to draw distinctions between them. Currently the rhetoric about working with communities implies, rather than defines, what approach is to be taken, and a mismatch between the conceptual approach and the desired outcome is one of the main reasons some processes in working with communities are ineffective.

The contributions approach is likely to be successful if communities of interest or of place are likely to gain a significant benefit from their contributions. Because of the need to achieve clear goals and targets within short timeframes, the instrumental approach is currently the dominant approach in Australia. Using this approach, there will always be a tension between the top-down planning process and the achievement of benefits from the community perspective. The empowerment approach is a central component in health promotion enabling people to increase control over, and improve, their health. It is also fundamental to community development. The developmental approach values the processes of achieving the task as well as the task achievement itself. In practice, the approaches are not discrete and are almost always found in combination. A developmental approach in working with communities of place or of interest has advantages, as it can lead both to task accomplishment and benefits for the community as a whole.

The approaches are often used in combination, and this is the preferred approach. A community empowerment approach will almost always be developmental. An instrumental approach may have some elements of a community empowerment approach. It is making the approaches explicit that is the most important factor. Then it is possible to ensure that all the strategies developed are consistent with the overall approach.

USEFUL WEBSITES

The Centre for Rural Health and Community Development undertakes research into approaches to community development:http://www.unisa.edu.au/cre/researchconsultancy/crhcd/default.asp

The Centre for Citizenship and Human Rights is concerned with issues of citizenship, human rights, community, civil society and social diversity: http://www.deakin.edu.au/arts/cchr/

CHAPTER 6

Practice Frameworks for Working with Communities

Introduction

Chapter 5 defined the four main conceptual approaches to working with communities to develop community health and wellbeing. These are the contributions, instrumental, community empowerment, and community development approaches. In addition, there are a number of practice frameworks that provide specific advice about how to develop community health and social care programs and initiatives through community work. This chapter presents five of these:

➤ interactional community development (Wilkinson 1991);
➤ participative development (Cohen and Uphoff 1977);
➤ building capable communities for health promotion (Labonte and Laverack 2001);
➤ building collective capacity in community-based programs (Moyer et al 1999); and
➤ asset-based community development (Kretzmann and McKnight 1993).

The frameworks presented are selected from the many available on the basis that they provide sufficient detail about the steps involved to enable them to be used in practice. Because they are summarised rather than presented in depth, it is important to follow up the references and websites in order to use them appropriately. All the skills that are presented in Part 3—community decision-making, partnerships, community leadership, community planning, and building knowledge—are essential in using these frameworks.

Practice frameworks for working with communities

TABLE 6.1   Practice frameworks for community health and social care development

Interactional community development (Wilkinson 1972, 1986, 1991; Sharp 2001)	Community development is defined as purposive, positive actions taken by people working together across community sectors in ways that people think will improve the community. It may be in expressing community interests or solving community problems. Task accomplishment has five phases, each addressing an action problem: creating awareness; organising sponsorship; decision-making about goals and strategies; resource mobilisation; and resource application.
Participative development (Cohen and Uphoff, 1977)	This framework presents the three components, the 'what', 'who', and 'how', which are seen as crucial to participative development. It also has a component about assessing the context of participation and evaluating the initiative.
Building capable communities for health promotion (Labonte and Laverack 2001; Laverack 2003)	This empowerment framework identifies nine operational domains in which to build capacity: participation; leadership; organisational structures; problem assessment; resource mobilisation; 'asking why?'; links with others; role of outside agents; and program management.
Building collective capacity in community-based programs (Moyer et al. 1999)	This model identifies four stages of collective capacity-building: identifying common ground; working cooperatively; working in partnership; and working across the community.
The Assets-Based Community Development (ABCD) (Kretzmann and McKnight 1993)	This approach to community development focuses on working with the community strengths and enhancing these by working from within the community—working from the 'inside-out'. The stages in the ABCD include community engagement, community asset assessment, and using strengths to create action.

Practice tip 6.1

There is not one framework that will meet all needs and be relevant in all situations. Think about the political and policy environment in which you are working and the outcomes required. You might need to choose aspects of several frameworks and put them together.

The interactional community development framework

The first framework presented is based in the developmental conceptual approach, and uses community interaction theory (Wilkinson 1991) which was discussed in Chapter 2. The framework is presented in Wilkinson's book, *The Community in Rural America* (1991), and has been added to by Bridger and Luloff (1999), Cheers and Luloff (2001), and Sharp (2001).

The empirical work to develop this framework was undertaken in rural communities where the small community size enables the communication, collaboration, partnerships, and integration processes to be studied.

Definition of community development

According to Wilkinson (1991), community development consists of local people working together across sectors and interest lines in the interests of community betterment. There are two key points in this definition. First, community work is purposive, with an end point in sight that people are working towards. Second, people understand that this end point will be in the whole community's interests rather than in the interests of a section of the community, or their own interests. In Wilkinson's definition of community development, interactions between people across community sectors are fundamental. It is not just one sector of the community aiming to solve a community problem; it is all sectors coming together to jointly address community issues.

The community development tasks

Wilkinson (1991) identifies five types of issues in the sequence of community development. These are: problems with awareness; effective organisation; decision-making; resource mobilisation; and resource application.

The first task is to create an awareness of the issue or problem across the community and not just within certain community sectors. This may be a time-consuming process, depending on the nature of the issue and the degree of community connectedness. Once this has been achieved, then actions must be coordinated and integrated across social fields or sectors through networks or organisations. Then, all those people and groups who need to be included should be given an opportunity to say how the task should be progressed. Once there is a common understanding of what needs to be done and how to do it, resources need to be mobilised. Wilkinson's view is that it is the people and their relationships that are the critical resources, and mobilisation involves building cohesion, encouraging participation, and developing leadership. Resource application is the final stage. This involves a process of building community structures, such as organisations and networks that enable people to come together. We described this process in Chapter 2 as building the community field. Resource application also means making decisions about priorities and using the resources judiciously, given the current and future demands.

Strengths of the framework

The framework is embedded in community interaction theory and research about how rural communities develop, and the structure and function of the community field. It focuses on building the interactions across the community that enable the community to come together to solve problems and express solidarity and identity. Therefore, it is useful in working in a community where there are divisions and separations between groups leading to factional community power networks. It provides a way of analysing these divisions and working with them to build cohesion. The framework is consistent with a developmental or community empowerment approach to working with communities.

CASE EXAMPLE 6.1

Using the interactional community development framework

Greyleaf is a bustling, sizeable, regional centre. As a tourist destination and an administrative centre with a defence base, it has a significant turnover of the population. It is acknowledged that the Greyleaf community is not one community, but made up of different groups. Groups are divided on the basis of employment (defence personal, government employees, and tourism industry personnel) and culture. The local organisations, structures, and networks reflect these divisions, and it is difficult to bring the disparate groups together to plan for the community as a whole. In terms of the community power structures, the tourist operators comprise the dominant group, as they are able to collectively influence local government about what development should be supported and what should not

There is an exception to this. The Health and Welfare Board has for many years involved people from diverse sectors and interest groups, and provides an avenue for debate of some of the most important issues that affect Greyleaf. For example, when a new industry was being proposed, the implications for economic, social, and health outcomes were hotly debated. Board members are aware of the complex interaction of the need for development and the related increased demands for public housing, transport, and health and human services. In addition, board members are cognisant of the groups that are marginalised with regard to uptake of services, and may become more so unless particular plans are put in place.

Under the new regional health and social service arrangements, the Board is to be amalgamated with three other Boards in surrounding towns to facilitate regional planning. This would bring together populations across the state, creating larger markets for service provision. There is a view that amalgamation with other regions might mean loss of services.

Think about it

➤ Using an interactional community development framework, explain why the Greyleaf Health and Welfare Board is important in community functioning.

➤ If you had as your task to facilitate the changes in the arrangements for the new Board, how could you approach this task using the interactional community development framework?

Practice tip 6.2

The interactional community development framework is useful when working to build social cohesion across community sectors is necessary in order to get joint action happening.

A framework for participative development

Cohen and Uphoff (1977) developed a comprehensive framework to be used by development agencies in undertaking agricultural development projects, primarily in rural communities in developing countries. It is empirically based through an analysis of the successes and failures of United Nations development projects in the 1950s and 60s. The key principles underpinning the framework have been adapted for use in health promotion (Eng et al. 1990). Participative development is defined as people's involvement in decision-making about what can be done and how, their involvement in implementing programs, and their sharing in the benefits of those programs.

The context, the 'what', 'who' and 'how' of participation, and evaluation

The framework analyses three components of participative development: 'what' development is about; 'who' is involved; and 'how' development is undertaken. In addition, a comprehensive assessment of the context of participation is recommended, as well as an evaluation of how participants are involved in the benefits of development.

The first step is an analysis of the contextual factors that may affect development. This stage is to be as comprehensive as possible, because it was noted that the context of participation had often been ignored by development agencies as they adapted a project from one setting to another. In the case of agricultural development, factors such as weather conditions and the availability of resources to participate are important. Political factors, such as the ideology around participation, and cultural and social factors, such as power structures, and the attitudes to authority that may impact on development, are all considered.

The 'what' of participative development considers the nature of the task and the relationships that are established between local residents and professionals that are necessary to achieve the task. In this framework, local people can initiate a project, define the task, and lead the processes in collaboration with professionals. If professionals define the task, then they should do so in consultation with the community, in order for local people's needs to be met.

The second component, the 'who' in participation, considers that local residents, local leaders, government, and foreign personnel with development agencies all should be involved. No assumptions are to be made that local people are a homogeneous group, and developers are to carefully explore the participation of appropriate people in considering the task to be achieved. The use of the adverb 'participative' emphasises the necessity for partnerships and collaboration in development.

The third component of the framework, the 'how', describes participative development as cyclical and interactive processes. Assessing where the initiative for participation comes from (either mostly from above or below), which inducements for participation are involved, whether participation is voluntary or coerced, and whether the structures of participation are formal or informal and individually focused is important. There is an emphasis on participative decision-making. Participative processes that are conflictual require expert facilitation and appropriate leadership to keep the development project on track.

The final component is evaluation, and this is one of the earliest attempts to develop comprehensive indicators and measures of rural development participation. Projects are evaluated according to local people's participation in the what, who, and how, and in the project benefits. The evaluation approach, with its focus on community benefit, is useful in evaluating both community health and social care development.

Strengths of the framework

The framework is empirically based and comprehensive. Its focus on agricultural development is not limiting if it is the elements of the framework rather than the examples that are kept in mind. It is useful when using a community empowerment or developmental approach to working with communities.

Activity 6.1

Using the participative development approach with the Greyleaf community

Return to Case example 6.1 about the Greyleaf Health and Welfare Board. Using a participative development framework, what do you think might be the important contextual factors that need to be considered in planning the development of a new amalgamated regional planning structure?

Practice tip 6.3

Getting communities involved in decision-making is much easier if it has been a partnership approach from the outset.

Building capable communities for health promotion[1]

The description of the framework for building a capable community is taken from Labonte and Laverack (2001) and Laverack (2003). Although designed for health promotion, this is a particularly useful and accessible framework, and worth considering in both community health and social care development. The framework offers an approach using nine domains to operationalise the goals of empowerment in the health-promotion context.

The nine domains for capacity-building

The nine domains that are important to assess and plan to develop community capacity are: community participation; leadership; organisational structures; problem assessment; resource mobilisation; 'asking why?'; links with others; the role of outside agents; and program management. The empowerment process engages with individuals and small groups, and links them with structures in order to increase an awareness of their situation and what is needed for improvement. The process is participatory and encourages the sharing and challenging of ideas.

The four phases of capacity-building

There are four phases to the process of capacity-building: a preparatory phase, including a working definition of empowerment; an assessment phase that examines each of the domains in the community; a strategic planning phase to identify how to strengthen each of the domains if necessary; and a follow-up phase during which progress is measured.

The strategic plan to develop the domains for each domain consists of:

➤ the assessment of the domain;
➤ the reasons for the assessment;
➤ how to improve capacity of the domain;
➤ the strategy that will be used; and
➤ the resources needed.

Strengths of the framework

The nine domains were categorised from a textual analysis of the health, social science, and education literature, and compared with the community development literature and the emerging literature on community capacity. Therefore, the framework should be able to be used in community capacity-building generally across disciplines. The framework is comprehensive, and there are helpful examples to illustrate how an assessment, strategic planning, and follow-up can be undertaken in each domain.

CASE EXAMPLE 6.2

Community empowerment in a community of interest

A community of interest had developed in a city area around the needs of people with an intellectual disability. A group of parents had worked hard to lobby government to provide adequate services for their children. They felt that if they didn't stand up for their children's needs, then no one would. Over the years, the parents had contributed their time, expertise and resources, and their efforts had resulted in improved services. The group had gathered momentum and increased numbers, and had a newsletter, regular meetings, and an office in a neighbourhood centre. Strong bonds had developed among some of the parents. The common element that brought people together was having a child or young adult with an intellectual disability and needing group support to advocate for better services. With some parents, this was the only thing they had in common, and interaction between people was limited to formal events. With others, friendships developed that were mutually supportive.

On occasions, there was a need to bring people together to comment upon government initiatives and proposed legislation. This became more and more difficult as special interest groups developed. There were few networks that could potentially include everybody. The people who participated in leadership roles were extremely busy, wore 'multiple hats', and some people felt left out. Rarely was there time to make considered responses to policymakers.

Think about it

➤ If you were a community health worker using a community empowerment approach, how would you ensure that parents had the opportunity to contribute to a proposal for changed service delivery arrangements for people with an intellectual disability?

Practice tip 6.4

Helping the community to question and analyse its issues is fundamental to using this approach.

Building collective capacity in community-based programs[2]

This framework was developed through an action research project engaging with a community to achieve a health goal, which was reducing the isolation of frail elderly adults. The model was clarified through discussion with academics and practitioners involved in different types of health-promotion programs.

Four stages of community capacity-building

The four-stage model describes how practitioners engage with communities to establish a community-based health program, and at the same time build capacity. The four stages of program implementation are: identifying common ground; working cooperatively; working in partnership; and working across the community. Each of these stages has specific goals and outcomes, and progress from one stage to another depends on the ability of the practitioner to engage with the community to extend its work. Movement also depends on the interest in the community in taking up the programs that are suggested.

Each stage of the model requires different levels of community engagement in the development of the health programs. Getting to know the community and the structures and programs already in place is the first stage. Making an offer to work cooperatively in some aspect of an existing health program or teaching new skills that the community requests is the second stage. This stage, if conducted successfully, results in community awareness that the practitioner has a specific agenda, but is also useful in meeting community needs. Once this acceptance has been achieved, it may be possible to work collaboratively on a project that is directly related to the practitioner's goal. The final stage involves networking with other organisations and individuals to embed the initiative in existing strategies to help ensure sustainability.

Strengths of the framework

The framework is based on the instrumental conceptual approach to community health and social care development. It is useful in health promotion and social care initiatives that are practitioner-driven rather than community-initiated. It shows the steps involved in a practitioner gaining acceptance in the community and implementing a program building on this acceptance. The framework was developed through practice-based action research, and could be modified for use in different communities with different target groups.

Activity 6.2

Using a capacity-building approach with a community of interest

Return to Case example 6.2. As a community health worker, your task is to implement a 'healthy eating' program with the community. Using the capacity-building approach outlined above, what would be your first task?

Practice tip 6.5

Always ensure that the community you are working with is able to achieve an aspect of its agenda as well as yours.

The Assets-Based Community Development approach[3]

The assets-based approach to community development (ABCD) is capacity- rather than deficit-based, and it is often called 'inside-out' development because of the focus on looking inwards at the community's strengths (McKnight and Kretzmann 2005). The ethos of 'inside-out' development fosters community members' control over the direction of development and the use of local resources or assets (Healy 2006, p. 254). There is a broad definition of assets, including financial resources, information, community members' expertise, and organisations and networks.

The stages of ABCD

The first step in the community development process is to engage with community members, and building relationships is fundamental in this process. Second, community assets are mapped according to the level of accessibility at the individual, associational, and organisational level. Deciding the level of accessibility involves assessing the assets that are within the community and under local control, those that are within the community but controlled externally, and the resources that are outside the neighbourhood and are controlled by outsiders. For example, a community asset within the community under community control is a locally managed neighbourhood centre. There are tools available from the Asset-Based Community Development Institute (see Useful Websites, p. 120) to audit community assets and the level of their accessibility.

The next step is to use the information gained through the audit to build community strengths in order to use assets to improve health and wellbeing. There is an emphasis on building community enterprises, for example a local café, to create local employment, and develop resources that will be within local control (Healy 2006, p. 254).

Strengths of the framework

Assessing assets that already exist but might have been overlooked or unrecognised is one of the strengths of this framework. There are also useful resources such as a community-building workbook to guide mobilising local assets.

Activity 6.3

The ABCD approach with a community of interest

Return to Case example 6.2. The community has decided it would like to develop a housing co-op. If you were a human services worker using an ABCD approach, how would you find out about the community's assets?

Practice tip 6.6

Working with a community will be that much easier if you start with the community's strengths.

Notes

1   See Laverack 1999, 2001, 2003; Labonte and Laverack 2001.
2   See Moyer et al. 1999.
3   See Kretzmann and McKnight 1993; McKnight and Kretzmann 2005.

SUMMARY

This chapter has presented five practice frameworks that are useful in community health and social care development. Two of these have been devised for community development: the interactional community development framework; and the framework for rural participative development. Both these frameworks are developmental in that they conceptualise development as an interactive and evolutionary process in which local people have an active role.

Two frameworks that have been used in health promotion have been presented: building capable communities for health promotion; and building collective capacity in community-based programs. The final framework, assets-based community development (ABCD), has been used in both health and social development. Each of these three approaches is embedded in a community empowerment approach, and Moyer and others' (1999) framework can be used in an instrumental approach where the practitioner is implementing a community-based intervention and it is not initially community-driven.

Each of these frameworks is presented as an overview. There is insufficient detail to enable a practitioner to use the framework without referring to the original reference or to a website. The point of providing the frameworks is to illustrate the steps involved in community health and social development, setting the scene for a discussion of practice skills in the next section.

USEFUL WEBSITES

The Asset-Based Community Development Institute: http://www.northwestern.edu/ipr/abcd.html

The Aspen Institute Community Building Resource Exchange: http://www.commbuild.org/

The International Association for Community Development: http://www.iacdglobal.org/

CHAPTER 7

Government Roles in Community Health and Social Care Development

Introduction

This is the final chapter in Part 2, which is about the conceptual approaches and frameworks for community health and social care development. This chapter focuses on the important role of governments at the local, state, and regional levels in facilitating health and human services programs and initiatives. Although there have been changes in the roles that governments take in this area, which are discussed in this chapter, they remain key players. Governments provide resources such as funding, and may work in partnership with communities, providing technical assistance, links to useful networks, and opportunities to develop policy.

This chapter presents information about two approaches. The first is community services development (CSD) (Williams 1996), a government approach to the development of social care initiatives that integrates policy development, planning, and funding with a developmental resourcing role in partnership with communities.

The second is community engagement, a largely government-led interaction designed to create greater involvement by citizens and communities in the development and implementation of government policies and programs (Cavaye 2000, 2005). Community engagement is currently a standard feature of Australian policies and institutional arrangements for implementing strategies in areas as diverse as the arts, community health development, social services, regional development, and natural resource management. It is also becoming apparent that the private sector, through the development industry and other resource industries, is increasingly involved in what it considers to be community engagement.

The two approaches, community engagement and CSD, are not discrete (Jan Williams, personal communication, 4 February 2007), as community engagement can be undertaken by the community with funding from government as another type of community-based 'service'. The community engagement service can then canvass a range of issues considered important by the community and in relation to issues where government thinks something needs to happen.

Government roles in health and social care development

Although the role of government in health and social care development in Australia has changed through public sector restructuring in the market state (Hancock 1999), it remains a critical factor. The question for policymakers in government currently is not whether government, contractors, the non-government sector, or for-profit organisations shall develop policy, and plan and deliver health and human services, but how all sectors will work together.

In some cases, communities of place and of interest require that governments play their part in service provision, as the community has not the capacity to do so alone. The reverse is also true. Previously, it was thought that if government was to provide the services, it did so in isolation. This is no longer the case, and decisions about how levels of governments and communities will collaborate should be important policy decisions.

Governments at all levels, nationally and internationally, have been promoting the benefits of government–community partnerships in health and social care development for at least two reasons. First, the complexity surrounding the provision of effective health and social care in the current climate necessitates joint problem-solving with communities to ensure appropriately targeted initiatives. This is especially true in the case of services for Indigenous people and those from culturally and linguistically diverse backgrounds.

Second, while government provides the necessary resources, including funding and technical assistance, and sets the policy framework, government can no longer control the implementation of initiatives. It must work with other agents, including communities, if there is to be effective implementation of policy.

Midgley (1986a, p. vii) argued that the position of the state in relation to community involvement in social development in Third World countries is critical, and can either hinder or facilitate social development:

> Since the state now dominates the lives and affairs of its citizens to an extent previously unknown, community participation advocates cannot ignore the activities of the state in social development. It is naïve to argue that state involvement in social development is superfluous and that communities in the Third World can solve the serious problems of poverty and deprivation wholly through their own efforts. While community participation is a desirable goal, the extensive involvement of the state in social development complicates the issue and requires further analysis.

Midgley et al. (1986b) describe four modes of state response to community participation: the anti-participatory mode; the manipulative mode; the incremental mode; and the participatory mode. In the anti-participative mode, the state suppresses community participation; while in the manipulative mode, support for community participation is for ulterior motives, one of which may be to reduce the costs of implementation or to enable greater political or social control of the community. The incremental mode is characterised by official support for participation, but a lack of, or ambivalent, support for it at the local level. In the participatory mode, the state approves of participation and resources it in a way that enables community members to take control of service developments through negotiations with governments, resulting in a powerful developmental process.

While Midgley's (1986b) typology remains useful, there is now a wealth of information about the participative roles that governments at all levels can take to facilitate health and social care development (Queensland Government/United Nations 2005), and a critical analysis of these roles, and the political context in which they take place, is timely.

In some cases, the impetus that leads to government involvement comes from a community. Sometimes it is government-led. In the example here, a local community approached local government for assistance in a health-improvement initiative.

CASE EXAMPLE 7.1

The healthy community initiative: Community and local government working together

The local health action group in a suburban neighbourhood approached local government to advocate for support for three health-improvement programs. These were a walking-to-school group, a Tai Chi group, and a display of healthy foods at the local supermarket. Local government was keen to assist, and sponsored a funding application to a national health-promotion program. It also offered to print a special edition of the local government newsletter on the initiative, and allocated some 'special purpose' funding. The local government representative with the health portfolio became a member of the action group.

Think about it

➤ What are the roles that local government took in this example?
➤ What are the benefits of local government involvement in this initiative?
➤ What might be the challenges of community and local government working together?

Practice tip 7.1

Always find out what leverage or power non-government organisations and communities can have in relation to government, and encourage the use of this power to advance the community's interests.

Community services development

Community services development (CSD) is an approach to the development of social care initiatives that makes explicit the respective roles of government and the non-government sector in providing a range of services and initiatives across sectors. Central to this approach is the belief that communities and non-government organisations (NGOs) have a capacity to deliver some human and health services, and that if they do, services will be more responsive to the diversity of client and community need. When we refer to the non-government sector, we mean all those non-government organisations, largely not-for-profit, providing health and human services programs. Philanthropic foundations, church social service organisations, and Aboriginal community-controlled health services are all examples of non-government organisations. Second, CSD is based on the principle that the process of developing services results in not only effective and responsive services but also in strengthening communities. The third principle is that CSD is a process that involves shaping government policy on the basis of practice experience. This case example identifies roles played by government in the neighbourhood centre.

CASE EXAMPLE 7.2

Identifying the roles government plays in the neighbourhood centre

The neighbourhood centre provides a range of services including information giving, has a telephone help line service, and coordinates volunteers for several agencies. It also provides meeting rooms for organisations and counselling agencies when they visit the neighbourhood. The centre receives funding from several government agencies to undertake these functions, and must meet accountability requirements for each program. These include financial reporting and different sets of statistics about service usage. Sometimes the centre has difficulty in complying with each of the funding programs' accountability requirements, and has developed a relationship with a government resource officer, who gives advice. The centre is also part of a government-funded national network that identifies emerging needs and priorities for human services delivery.

Think about it

➤ What roles do government agencies take in facilitating the work of the neighbourhood centre?

➤ What are the advantages of government involvement?

➤ What are the disadvantages?

Much of the information provided here about CSD is taken from the work of the Queensland Government and the NGOs who worked in partnership in developing practice and policy (Atkinson and Taylor 2000; Cruikshank and Darbyshire 2005; Felton et al. 1990; Williams 1993, 1996; Williams and Walsh 1994). A similar approach has been taken by the University of Washington in working with rural communities to develop community-based health services.

CASE EXAMPLE 7.3

Queensland Government Community Services Development

Source: Williams 1993

The 1990s was a period in which the Queensland Government initiated a comprehensive partnership approach between government and the non-government sector to identify and respond to community needs. The approach was premised on social justice principles that there should be equal access for all Queenslanders to appropriate services, and that the formal service responses should be contextually relevant and contribute to strengthening the community concerned. There was also an acceptance that there was a knowledge base and skill set that was necessary to successful community services development in order to ensure that activities strengthened the community.

The most important and defining feature of the CSD approach was that there was an interactive loop between the key processes of planning, funding, resourcing, monitoring and evaluation, and policy development. To implement this approach in an integrated way demanded considerable levels of reform within government and significant partnerships with the non-government sector, communities, and other levels of government.

Because of the necessity to link these elements, CSD practice was complex, dynamic, and continually evolving. It was developmental in that there was iteration between each element. The processes of working together were valued, and government consistently asked for feedback about how the processes could be improved. What was important to the success of CSD was that a degree of consistency of intent in government policy and practice was achieved over several years.

The four components of community service development

The following section outlines the four aspects of CSD: planning, funding and accountability, policy development, and resourcing.

Planning

CSD had social planning strategies in place, aimed at achieving an equitable distribution of resources across a region. It involved whole-of-government planning, where possible, to maximise the impact of responses to community problems. The focus of activities was upon rational outcome-oriented planning decisions rather than reactive and subjective responses to crisis situations. Planning was collaborative, with community and service provider input.

Funding for service provision was based on an annual collaborative planning process, with government, community, and service provider input that resulted in a State Plan (Queensland Department of Family Services and Aboriginal and Islander Affairs 1994–95).

Funding and accountability

Prior to the 1990s, government funding to communities and the non-government sector for social care initiatives used a submission-based model. The government

FIGURE 7.1   Community service development (CSD)

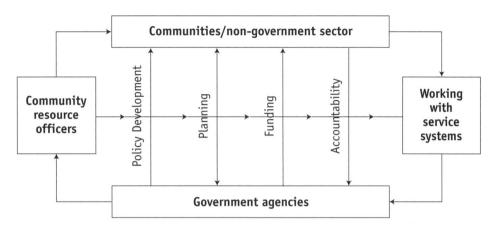

priorities were identified, the initiative advertised, applications sought and assessed, and funding allocated on the basis of the submission. The CSD approach emphasised a more equitable distribution of resources and the development of a planned approach to social infrastructure provision. Three factors were important in effective resource allocation: the spread of existing services; the adequacy of service responses to meet demand; and the capacity of organisations to provide. Qualitative and quantitative information was used to produce a profile for each of the regions. The resource allocation process used this information and made recommendations for funding against the three key criteria.

Accountability was required in both service delivery and the use of funds. The former was achieved by a service agreement developed between government and the NGO. This was a process driven by the program objectives and negotiated on an individual basis. Resource officers had a role in developing the service agreement and then monitoring it against performance outcomes. The use of funds was monitored by regular acquittals, an annual statement of expenditure, and audits.

Policy development

Policy development in CSD was an interactive process, with experiences of communities and organisations in developing and managing services informing policy in an interactive loop. Regional consultative committees were established to advise government agencies about issues and resolve them through negotiation. In addition, discussion with key stakeholders, communities, and government agencies contributed to policy development. The circulation of option papers was another strategy to engage communities and organisations in policy development.

As a result of this approach, CSD obtained a wealth of information about the service components that were clearly effective and those that were not. It enabled ongoing iterative information loops between services and government. Therefore systems and practices could be modified by input to policy development by people who had 'on-the-ground' knowledge.

Additionally, innovative funding and practice approaches to social issues were developed, most notably those that enabled holistic responses to community issues and services to Aboriginal and Torres Strait Islander communities (Queensland Department of Family Services and Aboriginal and Islander Affairs 1994).

Resourcing

The practice of CSD included a resourcing role to the community or NGO by government agency staff. It was acknowledged that financial grants to establish service responses should be accompanied by expert technical advice and developmental support by these staff. Some communities and organisations required minimal assistance, but where communities were less experienced, considerable support was provided. It was accepted that it was not cost-effective to delegate responsibility for service provision to a community without offering the necessary support and advice. The resource officer role was to ensure that the organisation provided an effective service, and in order to do this had access to the necessary skills and processes. However, the responsibility for financial accountability, as well as conformity to regulations and quality standards, remained with the organisation.

The resource staff had a dual role involving both monitoring the service's performance and providing technical advice and other support to service staff and management. The roles of regulation and support were performed concurrently, primarily through resource staff establishing appropriate relationships with the services staff and management. These relationships were the key to negotiating the roles when they conflicted.

Working with service systems

Another element of CSD was to work with service systems to develop effective service models. This was seen as a joint responsibility between the resource staff and the community and organisations concerned. In working with a service system, for example, services related to homelessness, the objectives might be to improve access and the referral processes. Identifying gaps in the service system was also important.

In this role, resource staff acted as facilitators and remained unaligned to a particular service. They built relationships between services, mediated different perceptions of roles and functions, and encouraged reflection about service activity. Case example 7.4 illustrates the planning, funding, resourcing, policy development, and working with systems roles involved in CSD.

CASE EXAMPLE 7.4

Family violence services development

Source: Felton et al. 1990

Several years ago, Aboriginal women came together from different regional areas in Australia to consult with government about the need for formal child care services. As part of this meeting, the problem of family violence was discussed. These issues were regarded so seriously by the women that on returning home, one of the women formed a women's group and wrote to government requesting support to build a women's safe house. Her request was referred to a government family violence program area. Government resource officers visited the location and met with the women and others in the community who were concerned about the problem. Over a period of a year, resource officers worked with women, organisations, local government, and the broader community to devise an appropriate service response. The women's group became incorporated, and resource officers put forward policy options that would enable the preferred service model to be funded. Additionally, resource officers contacted other government program areas that had an interest in developing Aboriginal health and wellbeing, and suggested complementary funding options.

Once the service was funded, resource officers assisted in the development of monitoring and financial management systems. While accountability for service functioning and financial management rested with the women's organisation, training in financial management, data collection, and evaluation was provided. Staff and community members associated with the service were supported to attend state and national network meetings to meet with other women involved in family violence services.

Think about it

➤ Why was government an important partner in developing this service response?

➤ What roles did the government resource staff play?

Practice tip 7.2

The roles of performance monitoring and providing technical support in service development need not necessarily conflict. However, up-front negotiation and clarification of roles is necessary.

Community engagement

This next section focuses on engagement of a community in the development of responsive government policy and practice. In health, it also involves increasing community participation in improving health. This is a generally a government or organisation-led process aiming to maximise involvement of communities of place or of interest in key issues. Community engagement practice in Australia and internationally has a raised profile in the face of accumulating economic and social changes, which have led to the catch-cry that 'governments are not listening' (Cavaye 2005).

Governments at all levels have become aware that, for the effective development of policies and the implementation of them, active involvement of stakeholders is essential. The term 'stakeholder' is used in the community engagement literature in a broad and inclusive sense to refer to any individual, group, or community, 'who has an interest in the issue, whether that interest is financial, moral, legal, community-based, direct or indirect... Any citizen or

CASE EXAMPLE 7.5

Community engagement to increase household recycling

A local government needed to increase household recycling and was about to approach its media unit to provide television advertising and radio broadcasts on the topic. One local councillor recommended a different approach—a community engagement strategy that had several components, including television and newspaper advertising. The first step was to hold a meeting including citizens, environmental groups, schools, and service organisations to get ideas and determine how everyone could be involved.

member of the public can be defined as a stakeholder if they have an interest in the subject being discussed' (Aslin and Brown 2004, p. 3).

The practice of community engagement has evolved largely intuitively to find ways to develop and maintain productive relationships between governments and organisations, communities, citizens, and clients. Currently, there is increasing dialogue to encourage the development of a body of knowledge and a set of skills that are relevant in the settings in which community engagement is practised. These settings are diverse and include health, performing arts, primary industry, local government, conservation, the environment, education, and Indigenous affairs. The International Conference on Engaging Communities conference website is a rich resource of information about community engagement theory and practice (http://www.engagingcommunities2005.org). Case example 7.5 is an example of a community engagement strategy initiated by local government.

Community engagement practice—two key aspects

Drawing on his wealth of experience with government engagement with communities, Cavaye (2005) defines two key aspects that define the nature of engagement practice: the level of engagement involved; and the extent to which the community, government or other organisations control and drive the process. Figure 7.2, adapted from Cavaye (2005), shows these two aspects.

Cavaye's (2005) integration of the level of community engagement with the degree to which community controls the process is a useful conceptual tool to analyse engagement processes. It is an advance on Arnstein's (1969) well-used ladder of citizen involvement because of its dual focus on the level of engagement

FIGURE 7.2   Levels and types of engagement in a healthy eating program

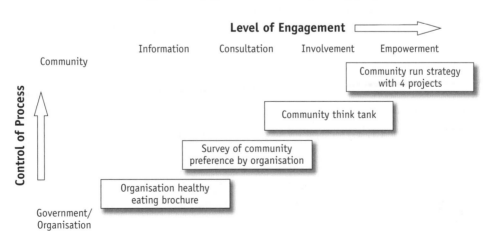

and the extent to which it is community-driven and controlled. Arnstein's ladder distinguishes six levels of citizen engagement. At the bottom of the ladder, citizens are manipulated by developers; then moving upwards, they have tokenistic involvement; then, they have some say in decisions; and at the top of the ladder, citizens have real power over decisions, and the process is community-driven. This framework has stood the test of time and is widely used, but it makes the assumption that planning processes will inevitably be driven externally.

While engagement practice always occurs in a political context, it need not always be driven by governments or organisations. In the current context, there is a tendency for all processes that are related to government's 'listening to the people' to be called 'community engagement'; for example, politicians meeting electors at country cabinets. It is possible that there might be a separate role for government to listen through its own independent processes. Community engagement could then involve a greater degree of community control. Cavaye's (2005) framework provides a useful tool to determine what level of government and community involvement is appropriate, given the task and the context.

First we will examine the four levels of engagement.

Levels of engagement

Cavaye's (2005) framework identifies four levels of engagement: information-giving; consultation; involvement; and empowerment. These levels are best understood as a continuum of increasing degrees of engagement. The first level, information-giving, is a very common engagement strategy and usually a pre-cursor to ongoing involvement. The importance of effective information to help plan for health and social issues is not to be underestimated. For example, one of the most serious issues in engagement of communities of place and of interest in health planning is the difficulty in providing de-identified information about the community's health status. Often the first step in community engagement is giving information about the topic in the form of a brochure or leaflet. The example in Figure 7.2 illustrating this level of involvement is a health organisation providing a brochure to community members to encourage a healthy diet.

Practice tip 7.3 Information-giving

For a range of health information resources for communities, see the National Health and Medical Research Council publication http://www.nhmrc.gov.au/news/media/rel06/givepub.pdf

The second level of engagement, consultation, is most effective when it is targeted, provides sufficient information prior to the consultation meeting, uses a realistic timeframe in which to obtain feedback, and gives information back to the community about the outcomes of consultation. There is considerable concern by communities about 'tokenism' in consultation, consulting when the government agenda is already determined, and 'over-consultation', which is continually revisiting communities with the same or similar topics. In the example illustrated in Figure 7.2, consultation occurs through the use of a survey to understand more about eating habits.

In Cavaye's (2005) framework, the third level 'involvement' describes an enabling rather than a directive approach, including forums and workshops intended to generate ideas and initiatives in partnership with government or agent. The involvement by groups, communities, citizens, and organisations inevitably has a capacity-building component in that the skills and resources needed to successfully implement a strategy are also discussed. In Figure 7.2, this level is shown through a think tank with community members and organisations participating.

Empowerment, as the fourth level of engagement, occurs when there is a sense of ownership of the strategy, a shared vision, the resources are in place for community leadership of it, and there are ongoing effective partnerships with government (Creyton et al. 2005). Figure 7.2 shows a number of strategies for healthy eating that the community will implement with assistance from government organisations.

Activity 7.1

Levels of community engagement —the recycling campaign

Return to Case example 7.5 about the local government strategy to increase household recycling. How and at what levels could the community be involved in the recycling campaign?

Degree to which the initiative is government- or community-driven and controlled

The degree to which engagement is government- or community-driven depends on the political context and the capacity of the community, as well as the nature of the issue involved. It is difficult for communities to drive the process when engagement is prompted by governments with a specific agenda. However, if governments want to find out feasible options for joint action, then community control is possible. This requires government agencies share information, advice, resources, expertise, and in-kind support. In any case, there must be a degree of reciprocity with some opportunity for community agendas to be met through the process if engagement is to be successful.

Usually there is a continuum of implementation from government initiation, to a partnership approach, and then to a community driving the process, which is illustrated in Figure 7.2. Even if government maintains control, at some point there must be a degree of government disengagement, and one option is government 'support from a distance'. This involves providing technical assistance on request or providing funding or other facilities to continue the initiative.

Activity 7.2

Who drives the process?

Return to Case example 7.5 about the local government strategy to increase household recycling. How could the community be involved in driving the community engagement strategy?

Principles of effective practice in community engagement

According to Moffatt (2005), whatever the level of engagement and the degree to which the community or government drives the process, there are key principles. These are equitable access to the engagement process, cultural appropriateness of engagement, appropriate staff, and appropriate methods.

Equitable access

Equitable access is about enabling people to get involved in consultation processes and other activities enabling a range of views and perspectives. Generally it is difficult to get involvement from groups that are marginalised in the community, and those who see themselves as 'outsiders'. There is a wealth of literature supporting sound practice in engaging 'hard to reach' individuals and groups (Cheers 1998, p. 149; Campbell and McLean 2002; Ife and Tesoriero 2006, p. 145), with one of the key factors being effective relationship-building. However, there are pragmatic concerns that may limit participation, such as limited resources, time, energy, and conflicting priorities. In small communities, people may put their time and resources into community engagement initiatives where they see the most return.

Practice tip 7.4

Engaging communities will only work where there is something to be gained from being engaged.

Cultural appropriateness of the engagement strategy

The engagement strategy must be designed with a sound understanding of the culture, values, and practices of the community that is to be engaged with. For example, in some Indigenous communities, it is inappropriate to have consultation sessions about men's issues with women present. In some regions, seasonal conditions can affect the schedule for consultation meetings. The wet season that affects the northern parts of Australia usually causes interruptions to road travel, and can isolate communities, making meeting attendance impossible. In Indigenous communities, it is important to understand that planned meetings will be inappropriate if there is Sorry Business occurring. (Sorry Business is a way of describing the grieving and mourning that occurs among Indigenous people as a result of a death.)

More than simply considering the timing or composition of meetings, the engagement strategy must consider all the unique cultural elements of the community of place or of interest that may have a bearing on the success of the strategy.

Appropriate staffing

The engagement strategy should also utilise appropriate staff. In culturally and linguistically diverse communities, it is essential to have a trusted member of the community introduce government personnel. In Indigenous communities, an Indigenous person who is considered appropriate by the group that is being consulted with should be involved. Government staff must have excellent communication skills and be able to negotiate different viewpoints. High-level skills in group facilitation will be necessary to ensure that the strategy is focused, conflict is negotiated rather than avoided, and groups and individuals are able to have their voice heard and listened to.

Appropriate methods

Much community engagement practice involves conducting meetings or workshops. The locations, style of the workshop, and timing, should be suitable to the community concerned. It may be helpful to schedule meetings to coincide with other events that are occurring in the community so as to maximise the opportunity for participation. Alternatively, if the meeting is at a location that will involve travel for participants, it is useful to plan meetings so that a number of purposes may be fulfilled. This case study is taken from a paper presented at the International Conference on Engaging Communities.

CASE EXAMPLE 7.6

Community engagement with women in the market garden industry

Source: Parker et al. 2005

Women from culturally and linguistically diverse (CALD) backgrounds working in the market garden industry in an urban fringe area had a need for information about occupational health and safety, including the safe use of pesticides. The women were socially and geographically isolated, worked long hours on the farms, and had childcare and household responsibilities in addition to their paid employment. Many had limited English language or literacy, and had restricted contact with industry organisations, which were the usual method of providing information and resources to the industry.

A government department made a grant available for an information strategy for CALD women in the market garden industry. The approach taken was to assist individuals gain information, but at the same time to learn about why access to information was difficult. This made it possible to give information in the context of women's experience and their values.

A small pilot project was undertaken with the Chinese community to provide accredited pesticide training. A bilingual Chinese woman who knew the farming community assisted with this and held an information session in the home of one of the participants, which was considered an appropriate location. The program gained legitimacy when women who had successfully completed training received their certificates at a community information day.

It proved more difficult to transfer the program to assist Cambodian women to access information. It was necessary to build personal relationships with the women to hear their stories and assess their need. However, there had been negative interactions between Cambodian farmers and government agencies, and many men were uncertain as to whether or not women should interact with government.

One of the ways to engage with these women was to provide English classes. Women were keen to learn English in order to be able to access services and interact more easily with others. The lessons built relationships and trust with the women, and enabled engagement with one section of the Cambodian community. To extend engagement, various strategies were used, including social activities, provision of technical advice, and computer training.

Strategies were successful because they were flexibly applied, acknowledged the women's experience, the diverse views in the communities, and most importantly they were built around social interaction among families.

Think about it

➤ Which of the principles of effective engagement—access, cultural appropriateness, appropriate staff, and appropriate methods—are illustrated in this case study?

Challenges in community engagement

As with all approaches to community involvement in government or organisational policy and planning, maintaining effective community engagement processes presents challenges for all. This chapter concludes with a discussion of four issues: engagement with communities when they are struggling with serious issues; maintaining continuity; balancing the government–community agendas; and engagement with CALD communities.

Involving struggling communities in future planning

The socio-economic circumstances of a community will determine the degree to which future planning is possible. For example, some Indigenous communities may exhibit high levels of concentrated and entrenched social and economic stress (Stark and McCullough 2005). These stresses result in people maintaining a focus on getting by on a daily basis, rather than getting involved in planning. The future is not a priority, and in many situations of extreme stress, the community and individuals are uncertain as to whether there is going to be a future (Wilkinson

2002). This is particularly an issue in Indigenous communities that are struggling to come to terms with the serious problems of economic and social disadvantage in addition to undertaking future planning (Felton et al. 1990). Therefore, it is essential to take into account the community history and plan a feasible strategy in consultation with the community.

Maintaining continuity

A second issue is the need for some engagement processes to extend over long periods of time, up to five years or longer in the case of some community renewal projects (Stark and McCullough 2005). Therefore, maintaining a consistent focus in the face of frequent changes of key personnel as well as changing government policy may make it difficult to maintain the integrity of the engagement. It is important to keep these issues of sustainability in focus throughout the strategy. Ensuring that there are viable local groups, spreading technical expertise and sharing information about all aspects of the project, may ensure that it can be sustained.

Balancing agendas

Inevitably there will be a requirement to negotiate competing agendas. For example, a government-driven engagement process may be directed to changing community health advisory structures. Communities may perceive that this will result in fewer opportunities for input to health planning. In this case, it is essential to use an enabling rather than a directive approach, and there must be time for communities to have their say and be listened to (Creyton et al. 2005). However, often government priorities necessitate tight timeframes for engagement processes. Personnel may believe a directive approach is necessary to keep consultation and information giving 'on track'. There is often a lack of knowledge about the community concerned and therefore a fear that the community will try to divert the direction of the engagement process.

This is a common problem in community engagement in health. Health planners usually assume that if communities or interest groups are given an opportunity to give advice about health needs and priorities, they may pressure

Practice tip 7.5

Practitioners need to make clear their organisational responsibilities and limitations, and at the same time enable communities to have a say.

for a level of service provision that is not feasible. This in turn leads planners to be wary of opportunities to engage with communities to identify pressing health issues and solve problems. There is a wealth of information now available for professionals to deal with this issue, particularly in health promotion (Moyer et al. 1999, p. 205).

Engaging with culturally and linguistically diverse communities

In engaging with these communities, it is essential to understand the cultural differences, and the impact that the different belief and knowledge systems will have on the engagement processes. The main strategy used by government to engage with CALD communities is through ethno-specific non-government organisations. Inevitably though, the community organisations that government seeks to work with will reflect the cultural perspective of its members, and not all individuals and groups will be represented. Those individuals and groups that are excluded may not be obvious to government agencies.

CASE EXAMPLE 7.7

Balancing community and government agenda

New government offices were to be built in a developing outer metropolitan area. Local government planners asked community groups to join a community engagement strategy to help identify the departments that should be represented, make suggestions about facilities, and advise on access issues. Most community groups did not regard the planned location for the building as suitable, and were unsure as to whether they wanted to get involved on this basis. It was difficult for the planners to engage with community members and groups because of this issue.

Think about it

➤ What strategies might encourage community groups to get involved?

➤ How could local government planners ensure that community groups had their say about the location?

➤ How could community groups obtain accurate information about the plan for the government offices?

Engagement with immigrants and refugees coming to Australia from diverse cultural and linguistically diverse backgrounds is of the utmost importance in reducing disadvantage. Arguably, many of these people are doubly disadvantaged due to their loss of employment, difference in skills base between country of origin and country of arrival, and lack of proficiency in the language of the country of arrival (Bagdas 2005). Therefore, engagement strategies will need to be informed by a sound knowledge of the issues involved. Case example 7.7 illustrates the need to balance competing agendas in community engagement strategies.

SUMMARY

This chapter focused on the roles that government can take in community health and social care development, and discussed two approaches. The first example is Community Services Development (CSD), which is an integrated approach to planning, funding, policy development, resourcing, and working with systems to create effective human services and programs. The second example is community engagement, which is a largely government-led interaction designed to create greater involvement by citizens and communities in the development and implementation of government policies and programs.

A key feature of the CSD approach is that it is underpinned by the belief that the non-government sector has the capacity to deliver some human and health services with appropriate support. Furthermore, CSD is regarded as an approach that will produce responsive services, but there will also be opportunities to strengthen communities. The third feature is that CSD is a process that involves shaping government policy on the basis of experience.

Community engagement is largely a government-led process aiming to maximise involvement of communities of place or of interest in a key issue, whether it be health planning, development of services or policy. There are four factors that need to be taken into account if an engagement strategy is to be successful. These are: ensuring equitable access; making the strategy culturally appropriate; ensuring that the strategy is appropriately staffed; and ensuring that it uses appropriate methods. There is a wealth of information available about how to conduct effective community engagement strategies, and the websites listed will put you in touch with this information.

Recent writing identifies that there are two factors that can vary in engagement strategies: the level of engagement with the community; and the extent to which it is a community or a government agency that drives the process. There were several issues in community engagement that were covered in this chapter including engaging with a community that is affected by serious economic and social wellbeing issues, maintaining the continuity and consistency of the strategy over a time period, balancing the agenda of the community with that of government agencies, and engaging with CALD communities of interest.

USEFUL WEBSITES

Community services development

The University of Washington community health services development home page provides information about the principles of working with communities to develop community-based health services: http://www.fammed. washington.edu/phc/test.html Accessed 30 Nov 2006

Community engagement

The International Conference on Engaging Communities conference website: http://www.engagingcommunities2005.org

The Queensland Government community engagement website: http://www. getinvolved.qld.gov.au

NSW Department of Infrastructure, Natural Resources and Planning Community Engagement Website: http://203.147.162.100/pia/engagement/index.htm Accessed Nov 30 2006

The Murray-Darling Basin community engagement toolkit: http://www.mdbc.gov. au/nrm/basin_communities/basin_people/community_engagement_toolkit

Skills in Working with Communities in Community Health and Social Care Development

Parts 1 and 2 presented information about the concepts, theory, and approaches that make up the framework for community health and social care development. Now we focus on the detail: the groups of skills that are used in all community work regardless of the discipline, whether or not we are community members or professionals, whether we are working with a community of interest or a community of place. The skill sets are related to:

➤ community decision-making;
➤ building and maintaining community partnerships;
➤ developing community leadership;
➤ community planning; and
➤ building knowledge about community health and social care development.

Chapters 8, 9, 10, 11, and 12 respectively deal with the skill sets related to each of these five aspects of working with communities. All of these skill sets will be used in every aspect of community work—they are generic. However, the type of development and the context in which we are working will mean that at times some are more relevant than others. Unfortunately, in community work there is no recipe for practice or when to use which skill sets. Each situation needs thinking through to decide what would work best and then applying the skills. This is why there are so many examples in Part 3 of typical situations that may be encountered. Discussing these examples with a group of people is the way to obtain different points of view about practice options. In some cases, check lists are provided that remind us of the key points that can be used in working with communities. At the end of each chapter are listed a number of Websites that provide helpful information for practice.

CHAPTER 8

Community Decision-making

Introduction

Community decision-making is discussed first because enabling communities to influence how programs and services are provided is fundamental to all other aspects of community work. However, this is one of the most challenging aspects. Facilitating decision-making processes that are collaborative, inclusive, and effective is something that no practitioner or community member gets right all of the time. The difficulty is in enabling people with diverse perspectives and with different values, attitudes, and priorities to have a say, and then negotiating how these views can be part of decision-making within tight timeframes.

Identifying the principles involved is essential, and then following some guidelines for maximising the chances of inclusive and collaborative processes is the next step. The other chapters in Part 3, on partnerships, leadership, planning and knowledge-building, all build on the information provided in this chapter.

The chapter presents key principles that support effective participative decision-making and information about community advisory groups and boards of management, which are typical structures to facilitate this. The steps involved conducting citizens' juries and charrettes are identified, and finally there is a discussion about decision-making in community-controlled organisations.

Some challenges of participative decision-making

The emphasis in this chapter is on participative decision-making, primarily between communities, practitioners, consultants, and government agencies. Inevitably, there are different agendas and priorities between these groups, and each has a power-base, which gives the group some ability to influence decision-making processes. Community people bring a range of skills, knowledge, and experience of the community and how it functions. Practitioners, consultants, professionals, and governments bring knowledge from their discipline, information about social and health issues, and money. The challenge is to blend community knowledge with that of practitioners, keeping within program guidelines to implement programs and services that are relevant and accessible.

It is acknowledged that community involvement in decision-making is difficult, and Warren (1970) noted that widespread involvement and efficiency in decision-making are in tension. The time taken to reach consensus, the difficulties involved in providing adequate information to inform the decisions, and the number of different interest groups wanting to influence the process, may make professionals very reluctant to allow community members to become involved.

Current policy on health and social care emphasises tightly targeted initiatives that require people with specialist skills to administer. If communities are involved, it is generally to promote and use the program once it has been planned. Practitioners usually define the context of decision-making, hold the power, and may be reluctant to transfer power in decision-making to community members (Stone, 1992, p. 412). Community involvement may be perceived as a threat to the power that practitioners have to 'keep the program on track'.

It is usually with the best of intentions that this pattern of control evolves. While at the heart of any kind of community development is the idea of change from below, this idea does not sit comfortably with top-down planning approaches focusing on quality and cost-effectiveness (Ife and Tesoriero 2006, p. 121). It is also a question of practitioners operating within a particular professional knowledge base and feeling most comfortable within this framework.

> [D]espite the aims of participatory approaches, and the claims made by participatory practitioners, particularly with respect to empowering the disempowered, it is argued here that participative methods of enquiry simplify the nature of power and are in danger of encouraging a reassertion of power and social control not only by certain individuals and groups but also of particular bodies of knowledge (Kothari 1999, p. 142).

There are other challenges to participative decision-making. There is evidence that it is increasingly difficult to get people to volunteer for management committees, attend planning sessions, and contribute to fundraising activities in some country towns in Australia (Taylor 2004). It may be that communities see involvement as too time-consuming and burdensome (Brownlea 1987). Health and social care policy involves complex, contentious, and ethically controversial decisions, which may be seen as the domain of governments or professionals, and in the case of health, medically trained experts (Butler et al. 1999). People may feel intimidated if the topic is complex or technical and think that they have nothing to contribute (Towle et al. 2003).

Finally, there may be scepticism that there is a genuine role for community members to participate in the decision-making process. One of the reasons for this might be a history of 'one-off' consultations about needs with a lengthy period between consultation and implementation of programs, with the result that communities are unable to see the links. In addition, organisations face constraints in providing relevant information to use as a basis for decision-making, and there is a lack of acceptance of communities' experience as an information source (Abelson et al. 2002).

Overcoming the barriers

None of these barriers is insurmountable if both the community and practitioners want to work together to make decisions about programs and services. It is important to ask about the barriers rather than just assume what they are. How often have we made decisions because we didn't want to 'bother' seemingly overstretched community members, and perhaps the topic was too difficult anyway? It is only our perception that the community is overstretched, or that the topic is too technical or complex for community involvement. We must check if this is the case.

Our research shows that communities involved in organising general practice services in rural Australia didn't regard the processes as overly technical or complicated, and they were involved in all aspects, including recruitment, organising a business model, fundraising, and governance. Rather than feeling overwhelmed, they were proud of their achievements and thought that the community benefited greatly from the general practice services. (Taylor et al. 2006b).

In this case, involvement in decision-making about how to recruit and retain general practitioners was crucial if the communities were to remain viable. The issues directly affected most community members. Being involved led to a sense of the community being able to be in control and deal with the problem. The result was a sense of ownership of the initiative and pride in the outcomes.

If the community can see benefit from involvement, can access appropriate information, has a supportive structure to assist, good facilitation, and practical tools, processes may work well. Good facilitation involves taking note of the key principles that support involvement of communities in decision-making. These are presented in the next section.

Key principles in decision-making with communities

The principles presented here were developed for regional planning and are adapted from the US Alliance for Regional Stewardship (Henton et al. 2001), which has a constructive set of principles and tools to promote public dialogue.

Recognising contextual factors that affect decision-making

Contextual influences shape how communities get involved in decision-making. From her research in four geographic communities in Canada, Abelson (2001), found three sets of contextual factors that affect community involvement in health decision-making: social structures and attributes; community values; and whether or not it is a contentious topic.

Social structures and attributes

Power structures and divisions between competing interests are an important contextual factor. All communities at some time will exhibit power structures, norms or values, traditions, and practices that are unjust and exclusionary. The practitioner should ascertain how power structures operate and whether they result in inequity, exclusion, and marginalisation of community groups or individuals. The facilitator will try to join with all groups rather than just the powerful or less powerful. This requires acknowledging power structures as a given rather than undermining them or working against them. In this way, the practitioner remains credible, and able to work with all factions, the powerful and powerless alike (Korten 1980, p. 482).

Practice tip 8.1

Consider the power networks in the community as a first step in thinking about inclusive decision-making. The types of power networks were explained in Chapter 2.

Community values

Some community values may assist involvement in decision-making. Strong and shared community values of 'the community taking action to preserve local identity' engendered broad-based community involvement in decision-making about health in a rural Canadian community (Abelson 2001). There are many examples of traditions of civic engagement in decision-making about community economic and social development. A feeling of community attachment and an interest in community wellbeing is often related to involvement in decision-making, particularly in rural communities (Brehm et al. 2004, p. 405).

Involvement in decision-making in some communities may be gendered; that is, it may be common practice for only men or only women to make decisions about some issues, or become members of organisations. This may relate to cultural, spiritual, or religious traditions and practices. Cultural and historical barriers to involvement in decision-making are diverse and again are related to different ethic backgrounds, experience, class, or professional differences. Some culturally and linguistically diverse (CALD) communities may regard requests to become involved in decision-making with suspicion as it has not been within their experience for this to occur (Parker et al. 2005; Van der Plaat and Barrett 2005).

Practice tip 8.2

Working closely with community members is essential to understand community values and culture.

The nature of the topic

Community action may be prompted when the community is threatened by unusual events (Tilley 1973). The threat provides a common goal necessitating collective action by people who otherwise may have few common interests. A risk to levels of existing service delivery, such as the closure of a local hospital, school or bank, for example, is clearly a reason for community members to act together to determine ways to try to overcome the problem. Case studies provide several examples of communities becoming involved in making decisions about health services to keep services in the community (Legge et al. 1996).

Even if there is no immediate threat, strong community norms of civic participation may ensure involvement in decision-making when a community issue is identified. On the other hand, some communities may take a more laid-back, wait-and-see approach, and be very reluctant to get involved in decision-making.

There are other contextual factors that may support community participation in decision-making. In psychology, for instance, research correlating demographic variables with measures of participation in community activities has found that variables relating to 'rootedness in the community', living in an area longer, intending to stay longer, and having more children were seen as factors related to participation (Wandersman et al. 1987). Being aware of the factors that may influence a community to get involved in decision-making is fundamental. The case example following shows some of these factors that influenced involvement in a mental health program.

CASE EXAMPLE 8.1

Assessing contextual influences

A community health worker was interested in running a men's mental health program in a farming community. The worker approached several community leaders to ascertain their views about whom to involve in making decisions about what type of program to run, and how to run it. The advice was that there had never been any success in getting men to attend information sessions about mental health issues as it was uncommon in this community to acknowledge mental health problems. It was thought that the general practitioner was the person who was approached when there was a problem.

Think about it

➤ What contextual factors should the worker take into account in planning with community members about how to provide a program?

Clarity about which decisions communities may make

The second important factor is to be clear about is why the community is to be involved and what capacity there is for the community to influence the process. It is wise to be cautionary, objective, and honest in discussing these issues with the community. If decisions about the overriding policy or service directions have already been made, then it is not only important to convey this, but also to identify aspects of the proposal that the community may influence.

In the practice task following, the city council, because of funding restrictions, has determined the site of a proposed child care centre and the number of places to be provided, but there are aspects that the community can influence.

Avoiding top-down talk

Practitioners are comfortable when they can use discipline-specific language to describe problems and issues that they have a mandate to address. It is common to hear the terms such as 'support', 'strategy', 'target group', and 'intervention' when practitioners are explaining a new proposal to community members. Community members are assigned roles such as 'consumers', 'patients', 'service users' or 'lay' people.

Activity 8.1

Making decisions about child care services

The city council in an urban suburb has agreed to fund the building of a child care centre to accommodate the needs of residents who are finding it increasingly difficult to access full-time child care places. A long process of convincing the city council of the need preceded the announcement that the centre would be built with an allocation of twenty full-time equivalent child care places. This was less than the residents were advocating for. In addition, the location of the centre has already been determined in order to make use of council-owned property, and it is not the location that community members preferred. Now the council is encouraging residents to be part of decision-making about the number of places that should be made available to the three age groups: babies up to one year, one to three-year-olds, and four to five-year-olds.

Your task is to address a meeting to encourage community members to continue to be involved, and help determine the number of places that should be allocated to the age groups. How would you go about this?

One way to hinder public dialogue is to treat it as a one-way, top-down communication. The use of the practitioners' frames of reference, definitions, and technical descriptions of issues and problems can produce a communication gap between practitioners and community members. This, in turn, can convey the message that it is the responsibility of professionals or experts alone, rather than in partnership, to solve the issue.

The skills involved in explaining complex problems and issues simply are considerable and rare, according to Bramson (2000). Essential to successfully

Activity 8.2

Preparing a presentation

Your task is to choose an issue in community-based health or social care that you understand well. Prepare a concise explanation of the issue for verbal presentation to a Parents and Friends meeting at a city primary school.

conveying a message is to first have a really good understanding of the issue, and to recognise, and accept, that others may not share your understanding. It also involves accepting responsibility for conveying the information in a way that invites participation.

Involving the community in naming and framing issues

In community health and social care development, practitioners may come to a community well versed in their perspective on the issue, and confident that they have the available evidence suggesting what would be an appropriate intervention to address it. They have named and framed the issue from their perspective. On the other hand, community members are unlikely to be of the one view about what the problem is and how it should be addressed. If a practitioner is leading program development, then it is important to put practitioners' views and plans on hold temporarily if community members are to be given an opportunity to influence decisions.

First, with facilitation, community members are encouraged to discuss an issue, name it from different perspectives, and include people who are most affected by the issue. The skills involved here are enabling multiple voices to be heard. This is difficult, particularly if the topic is sensitive and there are differing views. One way to do this is to continually interpret back to the community the different perspectives on the problem until there is some clarity about what all the different views are.

Once this has been achieved, it is time to come to some agreement about how the issue or problem is to be named, and information about how it might be dealt with can be provided. The community's experiential knowledge should be acknowledged as a valid information source.

Activity 8.3

Framing and reframing issues

Using the issue that you presented to the primary school Parents and Friends Association in Activity 8.2, what are some different perspectives on the issue that might be held by association members? How would you approach naming and framing the issue with members of the association?

Providing appropriate information and resources

The provision of information about issues in a succinct and understandable format is essential if community members are to be involved in naming and framing issues. In the past, communities rarely have had access to up-to-date information, but now organisations such as health planning units are making health outcome information and service usage data available not only to health professionals but also to community members. This is essential if community input into decision-making is to be well informed. It is a blend of community knowledge about what might work in the community with the best available quantitative and qualitative information about the issue provided by practitioners that will be most effective in decision-making.

Resources to support involvement are essential. These may include the time and cost involved in the preparation of information about the issue, the cost of a facilitator to conduct a planning event, payment of travel expenses to meetings,

Activity 8.4

Giving community groups information

Using the issue that you presented to the primary school Parents and Friends Association in Activity 8.2, where would you source information, for use by the Parents and Friends Association, about the options to deal with the issue? What resources might be needed to support the association's involvement in decision-making?

Practice tip 8.3

Try these websites for information about health issues. Include community people in collecting information.
http://www.cochrane.org/consumers/homepage.htm
http://www.healthinsite.gov.au

Try these websites for information about social issues
http://www.humanrights.gov.au/social_justice/az_index.html
http://www.livingisforeveryone.com.au/about_framework.php
http://www.acoss.org.au/Publications.aspx?displayID=1

or costs of child care while parents attend the meeting. Often the costs involved in communities participating in decision-making are considered as an afterthought and are inadequate. For example, the level of financial resources available for a new approach to community participation in programming in a Canadian health department did not match the government's rhetoric about its importance (Boyce 2002). It is important that the costs of community involvement are factored into budgets at the outset.

Creating a safe public space

Every public conversation about community health and social care issues involves a range of perspectives, values, opinions, and attitudes. It is quite likely that those people who perceive they hold different views from the majority will be reticent to present their views in public. They may not feel safe to share their stories or personal experiences in case they are not listened to or taken seriously by other community members.

Creating a safe place for discussion and decision-making involves feeling comfortable about the setting and the way people interact with each other. One way to do this is to let people have a choice about the setting where the discussion is held. Choosing a setting that people are familiar with, such as a neighbourhood or youth centre, may make participation easier. Providing child care, if appropriate, or transport for those who may require it, helps show that having people attend and contribute is important.

Helping people interact and share experiences and ideas is to have the meeting facilitated by an appropriate person in terms of age, gender, and cultural background. Using appropriate interpreters or facilities such as signing is important.

Activity 8.5

Creating a safe public space for decision-making

The members of the Parents and Friends Association usually hold their meetings at the school. Would this be an appropriate location for a meeting to discuss the health or social care issue you have chosen? What are some of the ways that you would ensure that all of the participants at your presentation (see Activity 8.2) might feel comfortable to enter into the discussion?

Organisational structures for decision-making

This next section provides information about organisational structures commonly used to support community involvement in decision-making; community advisory groups; and boards of management. Having the right structures in place to support decision-making is essential. Case studies of successful implementation of new methods of health service delivery found that viable health consultative structures were preconditions for success.

> In around 40% of our interview cases, institutional structures and policies (including legislation) which provided for or required community involvement in decision-making, appeared to constitute important pre-conditions for good practice. (Legge et al. 1996, p. 94)

Even if the structures are appropriate, this will not ensure effective decision-making. Professionals and communities must be willing to use the structures appropriately, and the bottom line is the extent to which professionals consider that communities have a legitimate role in making decisions (Baum and Kahssay 1999; Frankish et al. 2002).

Community advisory groups

Many programs and initiatives require a community advisory group to explore strategies, analyse issues, disseminate information, and make decisions. These groups have a variety of names and functions, but usually they involve community members from a wide cross-section of the community participating with practitioners and key stakeholders. The community may be a community of interest or of place. Community advisory groups have regular meetings, and usually there is a designated leader, facilitator, or chairperson of the group.

Is there an existing group?

Before creating a new group, it is important to check if there is an existing one that may be extended. Building on existing structures, rather than creating new ones, may be preferable. This is particularly an issue in small communities where there may be a proliferation of committees attached to each different program or interest area. Community members become overburdened, may be placed in conflicting situations regarding competing needs and priorities of the groups, and may wear too many 'different hats' (Baum and Kahssay 1999; Jacobs and Price 2003).

Existing groups associated with schools, the environment, community development, health, or youth issues may be an appropriate auspice. These groups may have an accepted place in community life, an existing membership, and mechanisms for decision-making. While the membership of existing groups may not be sufficiently diverse, it is worth considering how the group could be expanded to make it more appropriate. Building new structures may undermine existing ones, and the decisions made by the new group may not be seen to have credibility.

Activity 8.6

Establishing community advisory groups

A new program involving education and training for community groups in suicide prevention is to operate in a city suburb. The funding guidelines for the program require a community advisory group to be established to make decisions about what training to run and who should be involved. Consider what factors you would take into account in deciding whether to look for an existing organisation to sponsor this advisory group, or to develop a new one.

Practice tip 8.4

Look broadly for an appropriate structure for a community advisory group. Consider sporting clubs, leisure centres, service organisations, and universities.

Getting members

Participant selection is a major consideration in establishing decision-making structures such as community advisory groups (Abelson and Lomas 1996, p. 49). In health and social care, people volunteer for boards and advisory groups because they have specific technical or management skills or because they are interested in the issue. If they are selected through some formal process, it is often because they are knowledgeable about the diversity of the needs of groups of actual or potential users of services, and can represent those needs. This is known as 'representative participation'.

What constitutes representative participation has been the topic of considerable debate (Abelson 2001; Baum et al. 1997, Baum and Kahssay 1999; Milewa et al. 1999). There is an expectation that participatory structures will be representative of the range of community members. If particular groups, for example young adults, gay or lesbian groups, or older adults, are not represented, then advisory structures may be considered to be unrepresentative. This argument may be critiqued on two counts.

First, the idea of achieving genuine representativeness, or a person being able to represent all the needs in the community or even those of a particular subpopulation, is never feasible. Advisory structures can never become a 'microcosm' of the population as a whole, reflecting the different views of all the groups in the community. Second, the involvement of even a few local people ensures more local input into planning than would otherwise be the case even if the views they express are not 'representative' views—that is, they do not represent all the views. This is because 'being representative' and 'representing' are different things. Research in rural areas in New Zealand and Canada found that members of advisory structures regarded themselves as 'representing' community values and the local identity of the community in which they were members as they contributed to decision-making. They were community members and therefore they were 'representing' community (Abelson 2001; Eyre and Gauld 2003).

It is important to be explicit about the reasons people are selected to participate in decision-making. Is it that a range of community perspectives is important, or is it certain types of views?

Practice tip 8.5

Pragmatically, it may be impossible to balance skills, perspectives, and experience when calling for membership of a community advisory committee. Participation of people with an interest in the topic and energy to contribute may be an appropriate option.

Community advisory group roles and responsibilities

Community advisory groups should have clear and time-limited objectives, and members should have identified roles and responsibilities. People should be well aware of why they are on the community advisory group and what they can contribute. Working towards the objectives of the group must be of value to all those involved, and there must be relevant incentives to support participation.

CASE EXAMPLE 8.2

The Disability Forum

The Disability Forum in an urban location was established by the city council to provide an opportunity for community input into policy and services for people with a disability. It has a stable membership of people with disabilities and their carers, professionals working in the area, local government representatives, and interested community members.

While the concept of the forum was enthusiastically received by the disability community, people were unclear about the influence the forum could have with the city council. Therefore the city council and members of the forum together drafted terms of reference for the operation of the forum. These included the objectives of the group, membership, and decision-making processes.

The council appointed a facilitator to assist discussion about issues and to enable different viewpoints to be included in the decision-making processes. Where the forum has been able to reach agreement on issues, there is a process for recommendations to be made to council meetings where the final decisions are made.

One of the difficulties the forum has is how to include minority views in the council's deliberations. The topics under discussion are often complex, and there are diverse viewpoints. The experience has been that sometimes it is not possible to reach agreement.

Think about it

➤ What factors about the forum would support effective decision-making about policy and services?
➤ What would be some of the limitations of this structure in effective decision-making?

There should be clear processes for decision-making (Cruickshank and Darbyshire 2005). Case example 8.2 shows how this can occur.

Boards of management

Many hospitals, health services, and community service organisations are formally incorporated, or established through legislation, to take responsibility

Practice tip 8.6

Check list for setting up community advisory groups (adapted from the *Community Development Tool Kit* (Edmonds 2005): http://www.engaging communities2005.org/abstracts/S117-edmonds-lf.html

- ➤ Is there an existing group that is appropriate?
- ➤ What structures are needed for effective decision-making?
- ➤ How many members are needed?
- ➤ How will members be chosen?
- ➤ Will there be a facilitator?
- ➤ How will decisions be circulated?

for organisational governance functions, including financial management, quality assurance, and planning. There are designated positions such as 'chairperson', 'vice-chairperson', 'finance manager', and 'general member'. Finance and planning is conducted through subcommittees of the board.

CASE EXAMPLE 8.3

The Social Care Board

The board of a large social care organisation has a long history in providing innovative health and social care services in the city and in regional centres. Its services include family counselling, accommodation, and disability services. The board has members from the church that auspices the organisation, members with technical skills, and representation from staff, volunteers and service users. Originally the organisation was entirely city-based. Now regional service delivery is an important part of the organisation's role, and board members think that decisions should be informed by a regional perspective. However, there are no places on the board for regional representatives, and logistically this would be difficult as there are frequent board meetings. Regional representatives would have to travel long distances to attend meetings.

Think about it

- ➤ How could the Social Care Board members obtain a regional perspective in making decisions?

Membership

Membership of boards is through election, in accordance with the constitution, although some positions may be available for specific groups, such as consumer representatives. Several of the organisation's staff may sit on the board, and may or may not have voting rights. Decisions are made through formal processes, including taking a vote, and decisions are minuted and circulated to members and the community more broadly. Information is provided prior to the meeting in relation to each of the topics for discussion. The same issues about representation apply to boards as in community advisory groups. Case example 8.3 shows how it is necessary to continually review membership to include relevant views.

Practice tip 8.7

Checklist for decision-making with boards of management adapted from the community development tool kit (Edmonds and Anglin 2005).

1. Plan for decision-making:
   ➤ Have written roles and responsibilities for board members in decision-making.
   ➤ Circulate concise information about the topics needing decisions ahead of time.
   ➤ Put forward options.
   ➤ Encourage transparency in decision-making.
   ➤ Keep an accurate record of decisions.

2. Encourage efficient committee work:
   ➤ Establish subcommittees for some topics.
   ➤ Ensure clarity about which decisions are made by the sub-committee.
   ➤ Ensure there is effective information flowback to the board.
   ➤ Ensure membership is appropriate to the task.
   ➤ Ensure members are not overloaded.

Techniques for community involvement in decision-making

This final section of the chapter provides information about techniques for community involvement in decision-making. There are a number of websites that provide information, and these are listed at the end of the chapter.

Citizens' juries

Citizens' juries are commissioned by a government agency or an organisation to assist decision-making about an issue. All the processes involved in selecting participants, disseminating information, and making recommendations are transparent. The method has been used to make decisions in planning and conservation, and is beginning to be used in health care provision. In health, Mooney and Blackwell (2004) found that prioritising health needs in the context of community values was very effective, more effective perhaps than engaging with consumer groups, who tend to prioritise their own needs. The benefit of citizens' juries is that they will enable judgments to be made about issues that are of importance across the whole community and affect everyone. They may be used to make recommendations about an issue from a prepared set of options.

For further information, see URP Toolbox: https://www3.secure.griffith.edu.au/03/toolbox

The format of a citizens' jury

Participants are chosen on the basis that they are members of a community of interest, or of place, rather than because they have particular knowledge of the issue. One sampling method is to draw participant names from a telephone book, or the electoral roll, and then send invitations through the mail. Replies to the invitation can be stratified on the basis of age, gender, or length of residency, or other factors to reflect the demographic composition of the community. It is usual for juries to consist of between eight and twelve members.

Practice tip 8.8

Check list for decision-making using a citizens' jury:

- ➤ Is the topic suitable for a citizens' jury?
- ➤ How will jurors be chosen?
- ➤ Which experts will be involved in providing information?
- ➤ Who will moderate the provision of, and discussion about the information?
- ➤ How long will the jury have to come to a recommendation?
- ➤ Who will moderate this process?
- ➤ To whom will the report be presented?
- ➤ How will jurors be told about the uptake of their recommendations?

CASE EXAMPLE 8.4

The health priorities citizens' jury

Source: Mooney and Blackwell 2004, p. 76

The citizens' jury was to determine a set of priorities that jurors thought were most important in the context of limited resources. Jurors were requested to take a community focus and make decisions for the whole community, not just themselves as individuals. Jurors were chosen randomly from the electoral role, presented with balanced evidence, and given time to discuss and deliberate with a facilitator. The jury was able to identify and debate issues of broad principle, such as equity, when referring to community values.

Think about it

➤ What is the value of the citizens' jury in determining health priorities?
➤ What are the differences between engaging with health consumer groups and engaging with communities to determine health priorities?

The format involves an adequate preparation for jurors through presentation of technical or demographic information, as well as community perspectives relevant to the deliberations. These experts spend time discussing the issue with the jury and can be cross-questioned. If appropriate, a visit to observe the issue is included in the preparation. Jurors are also briefed on the rules of the proceedings.

An independent moderator assists the jury in the process of deliberation, which may take up to two days, and the jury makes a judgment in the form of a report containing its recommendations. Usually, assistance is provided to record the discussion and in the preparation of the report. The organisation that commissions the jury responds to the recommendations, follows them, or explains why it did not. Case example 8.4 is an example of a citizens' jury.

Charrette

The charrette is a structured presentation of plans, options, and ideas, held over several days to enable intensive discussion, brainstorming, and decision-making with communities about a proposal or an issue. It is frequently used in planning. A display is constructed, usually on site, using a variety of media, such as videos, models, and photographs, to illustrate the issue or proposal. Interest groups, community members, and key stakeholders are encouraged to review, comment upon, and make decisions.

The charrette provides an opportunity to bring together community members, experts and practitioners who have an interest in the issue and who can contribute to decision-making. It provides a heightened focus on the issue and rapid and dynamic interchange of ideas between planning practitioners, stakeholders, and the general community. It is a cost-effective means of envisioning the outcomes at an early stage, and assessing the proposals at the final stage. It can be used to launch a project, celebrate completion, or to demonstrate the options at a significant choice point.

An effective charrette is resource-intensive. It requires bringing experts and community members together with sufficient time for adequate discussion. The cost involved in preparing the visual material may be considerable.

CASE EXAMPLE 8.5

An urban renewal program

An urban renewal program funded by two levels of government held a charrette to display and make decisions about the style of housing and public space options to be used in the renewal. The event was held over two days at the community information centre. Local volunteers, community members, and local government staff were involved in organising, facilitating, and evaluating the event. Planners contributed models, sketches, and video presentations about the renewal options. Regular timeslots were allocated for decision-making, and careful facilitation occurred to support this. Plans were made about how community members might continue to be involved.

A highlight of the event was the visual presentation by community members of the places that represented what they valued in the community, and how these might be developed. An evaluation of the event was conducted, and several working groups were established with local involvement.

Think about it

➤ What was the value of the charrette in decision-making about urban renewal options?

➤ Which factors about the planning of the charrette supported involvement in decision-making?

Practice tip 8.9

Decision-making using a charrette:

➤ Is the topic suitable for conducting a charrette to make decisions?
➤ Where will the charrette be held?
➤ Which resources are required and who will develop them?
➤ How will decisions be made about the topic?
➤ Who will be involved in making decisions?
➤ How will decisions be communicated and to whom?

Decision-making, community control, and community ownership

This section is about the role that is played by community-based organisations in community health and social care development. We examine this from the perspective of decision-making and what is meant by 'community control'. We are also interested in the relationship between community-based organisations and a sense of community ownership of these organisations. The connections between community control, involvement in decision-making about services and a resultant sense of ownership, and increased usage is complex. It is important that further work be undertaken, at the community level, to explore these relationships. First, it is important to examine the role of the non-government sector.

The non-government sector

Community-controlled organisations are part of the non-government or Third Sector. The non-government sector, in the context of health and human service delivery, comprises those non-profit organisations governed by a management board or committee established to meet specific service delivery needs. In social care provision, there are numbers of these organisations providing a wide range of services, including accommodation, child care, and information.

In health, there are men's health services, health information services, disability services, and mental health services that are non-government organisations (NGOs). Aboriginal community-controlled health services are a common example of a health NGO. There are more than 140 of these in cities and regional, rural, and remote towns in Australia (Bell et al. 2000). These have been established because of the failure of mainstream health services to meet the needs of

Aboriginal people, and because of policy moves towards self-determination and self-management (Franklin and White, 1991).

Currently, the non-government or Third Sector has a central role in community health and social care development, and should, according to Lyons, (2000 p. 184) be given more recognition by government. Historically, the non-government sector's role was service provision in areas where government could not or would not participate. There are many examples of children's residential facilities and disability services being established by NGOs. Now the majority of organisations that make up the human services and health non-government sectors are not-for-profit, and their intention is to provide services for public benefit, primarily through the utilisation of government funding.

NGOs have an increasingly important role in community health and social care development. They can provide services using funding from sources other than government, including philanthropic trusts and foundations, and this makes it possible to innovate. Second, most non-government organisations have a role in advocacy for the client groups they serve and have overarching or peak organisations to lobby and participate with governments in policy development. The Australian Council of Social Service (ACOSS), for example, leads and supports initiatives within the community services and welfare sector, and acts as an independent non-party political voice. By drawing on expertise of its

CASE EXAMPLE 8.6

Panthers on the Prowl Community Development Foundation

The Panthers on the Prowl Community Development Foundation operates autonomously under the auspice of the Board of the Panthers Rugby League Football Club. Richard explains the organisation's role.

> Basically, we see it as our function to build capacity in the community, which includes building neighbourhood social cohesion. Probably, there has been a change of culture here to have a sports centre turn to a community focus, but we all acknowledge that the community exists beyond the stadium and is bigger than the football community. We all believe that we have to give back to our community, and we had a Board looking for opportunities to do this—how to make this region a better place.

We have programs, government funded and with strong support from the licensed club, with our school communities involving an active lifestyles initiative, programs for students at risk of disengaging from the learning process, a teacher's aide mentor program, and a parent support program. For example, our School Community Support Program provides a classroom here in the sports stadium, with a state-funded teacher who is with selected children taken from their regular school in the mid morning and back in the afternoon. The program aims to build resilience, literacy, and social skills. The parent (family skills) program provides a forum for group discussion. We believe that parents need to have a range of opportunities to meet and form supportive relationships with other parents.

Opportunities to build social capital in our community continually spin off—we work through the schools in our region, as we have strong relationships there, and then that links us to parents who we work with as well. So much community work is communities having things done to them rather than with them. Often things are started and then stopped when the money runs out. We are on about building sustainability. For example, to get parents involved beyond the family skills sessions, we held a morning tea group discussion in the chairman's lounge and asked them if they would like to continue facilitating this type of group. They agreed, and then we step back and provide moral and material support rather than hands on. Other opportunities present, which enable us to provide funding and material support to other organisations.

One of our key strategic pillars is to develop the cross sector relationships with other NGOs. Often NGOs don't talk to each other, and we need to get beyond the 'turf' disagreements. We are able to provide a venue to get NGOs together to build face-to-face relationships, and we have been involved in joint activities with key organisations in our district.

Evaluation drives our programs and it is important to seek out opportunities to evaluate. If we evaluate well, and we are following up our students after the program ends, then the program becomes student and parent led. We need good strategic plans, structures, and processes in place and good data to understand how and where we are going. We need to be conscious of the fact that we are dealing with public money and use funds to maximise outcomes by refining what we do on a regular basis.

For more information about the Panthers on the Prowl programs, go to their website
http://www.panthers.com.au/default.aspx?id=71

diverse member base, ACOSS develops and promotes socially and economically responsible public policy and action by government, community, and business.

Case example 8.6 provided by Richard Booth, Manager Educational Programs, Panthers on the Prowl Community Development Foundation, demonstrates how an innovative NGO can help develop health and social care in its region and encourage NGO sector linkages.

Decision-making in community-controlled organisations

Community-controlled agencies are likely to have existing relationships with community members, have up-to-date information about community issues, needs and competing priorities, and be aware of community perspectives. Because of their relationships, they may be able to involve relevant people in decision-making quickly, and this is very useful when timelines are tight. They may have experience of what works best in the local context.

On the other hand, community-controlled organisations may represent sectional interests rather than the community as a whole. Alternatively, decision-making may not be transparent, with only a small group of the organisation taking part. It may be difficult to encourage sufficient people to be part of management committees to make decisions, and this is always a problem in small communities of place or of interest.

The following is an example of a community-controlled service and how they make decisions.

CASE EXAMPLE 8.7

The Youth Shelter

The Youth Shelter, in a regional centre, provides accommodation, counselling and a work cooperative for homeless young men and women. It is run by a community-based organisation that has a management committee of twelve members. Membership of the committee is diverse, with a gender balance and people of different age-groups and cultural backgrounds. The Anglican Church originally sponsored the organisation and there are several church members on the committee. People join the management committee because of their strong commitment to the issue of youth homelessness. A commitment to volunteering for various tasks at the shelter is involved in order that members gain a sound understanding of the issues young people experience.

Decision-making about service directions involves input from the management committee members, young people, and the shelter staff. The management committee meets monthly and uses everyone's input into decisions. There are regular events, such as evening meals, at the shelter where the residents and management committee members can meet each other informally and discuss issues. In this way, residents can also have a say.

Community control and ownership

It is likely that where there is strong community decision-making in developing services and programs, then there will be a sense of ownership of them. Where there is a sense of ownership, it is possible that the services will be relevant and accessible. This is the case with Aboriginal community-controlled health services.

In country communities in Australia, hospitals and general practice services are highly regarded because of the need to access services locally, and because of their contributions to community viability. There is often a sense of ownership of the services.

CASE EXAMPLE 8.8

In Our Hands Health Centre

The In Our Hands Health Centre is a drop-in health information and resource centre for the whole community. It is run entirely by fully trained volunteers, and provides health-related information in various formats, including advice, Internet access, brochures, and courses. Its focus is on assisting people get the most out of life when living with a chronic condition. The centre is located in a shopping centre and provides a base for a number of support groups. The centre is now a fully incorporated body with its own management committee, made up of eight elected volunteers and four non-elected positions, which are filled by local health-related partners. Networking with health service providers (local, state, and federal) plays an important role in the centre's future, as without their support and input, it could not work as effectively as it does currently. For more information about the In Our Hands Health Centre, go to the website http://www.inourhands.com.au

As a community member I see myself as owning the health centre and so this means to me that we have to support it. If we want to retain our services then we need to do whatever we can to help the doctors whether it is just moral support, friendship, fundraising, or sitting on the board. (Taylor et al. 2006b, p. 146)

Case example 8.8 is an example of a community-initiated health service, In Our Hands Health Information and Resource Centre, Whyalla, South Australia, which provides a range of health information and activities for community members. Community members are now involved in all aspects of the centre's functioning, and therefore there is a strong sense of community ownership. People who volunteer at the centre and those who use it value the service and work to ensure it continues.

SUMMARY

This chapter has provided the key principles that support effective community involvement in decision-making:

➤ recognising contextual issues that affect decision-making;
➤ avoiding top-down talk;
➤ involving community in naming and framing issues;
➤ creating a safe public space;
➤ providing appropriate information; and
➤ providing appropriate resources.

The key issues in creating structures to support decision-making were discussed, including how to choose participants and when to use existing organisations' structures, and when to create new ones. Two structures for decision-making were discussed, community advisory committees and boards of management; and two decision-making techniques, citizens' juries and charrettes. The non-government sector and community-controlled organisations were discussed with regard to decision-making processes, and the relationship between community involvement in decision-making and a sense of ownership of the services.

USEFUL WEBSITES

Resources for decision-making

The URP toolbox is a source of information about tools for working with communities. It was developed by the Coastal Cooperative Research Centre: https://www3.secure.griffith.edu.au/03/toolbox

The Community Tool Box—a useful resource for specific skills in community work:
http://ctb.ku.edu
Techniques from the NSW Department of Infrastructure, Natural Resources and
Planning: http://203.147.162.100/pia/engagement/techniques/index.htm
A Framework and Toolkit to Work towards Whole of Community Engagement:
http://www.engagingcommunities2005.org/abstracts/S119-aslin-hj.html
Tool kit for community development and setting up a community organisation:
http://www.engagingcommunities2005.org/abstracts/S117-edmonds-lf.html
Citizens' jury—A case study about a Far North Queensland citizens' jury project:
http://cjp.anu.edu.au/simon/index.htm
Charette—iPlan Department of Infrastructure, Planning and Natural Resources
NSW: http://203.147.162.100/pia/engagement/techniques/charette.htm

Resources about the non-government sector

Australian and New Zealand Third Sector Research network: http://www.anztsr.org.au
Australian Council of Social Service—an example of a peak non-government
organisation: http://www.acoss.org.au
Aboriginal Health Council of SA—an example of a peak health organisation:
http://www.ahcsa.org.au/?page_id=28
The Panthers on the Prowl Community Development Foundation—an example of an
NGO: http://www.panthers.com.au/default.aspx?id=71
Pika Wiya Aboriginal Health Service—an example of a community-controlled health
service: http://www.pikawiya.com.au
In Our Hands Health Information and Resource Centre: www.inourhands.com.au

Resources for community organisations

Queensland Government Community Door—a one-stop shop for information and
resources for community organisations: http://www.qld.gov.au/ngo

CHAPTER 9

Community Partnerships

Introduction

Community decision-making was discussed in the previous chapter as one of the most important and challenging aspects of working with communities. This chapter builds on that information to discuss how to facilitate partnerships that are collaborative, inclusive, and effective—all the components that are important in decision-making. So again, a common theme will be evident—the importance of working relationships.

The focus in this chapter is on partnerships between communities, organisations, consultants, and practitioners that are intended to assist in health and social care development. The key principles underpinning successful partnerships are discussed, and two types of community partnerships are explored—horizontal partnerships between community sectors and groups, and vertical partnerships between communities and external agencies. Finally, the skills involved in the different stages of partnership functioning are identified.

Defining our terms

The terms 'collaboration', 'partnerships', 'linkages', and 'coalitions' are used similarly and even interchangeably in health and social care. Although there are no universally agreed upon definitions, there is an emphasis on a partnership, collaboration, or coalition as joint action to achieve mutually agreed upon goals. In health promotion, for example, the term 'community coalition' is used to describe an organisation of diverse interest groups that combine their material and human resources to effect a specific change that members are unable to achieve independently (Brown 1984, p. 4). A partnership is defined as 'an alliance among people and organisations from multiple sectors ... working together to achieve a common purpose' (Himmelman 1992, p. 74). Partnerships are defined similarly in business, as 'purposive strategic relationships between independent firms who share compatible goals, strive for mutual benefit, and acknowledge a high level of mutual interdependence. Firms join efforts to achieve goals that each firm, acting alone, could not attain easily' (Mohr and Spekman, 1994, p. 135).

Why establish partnerships?

The emphasis on partnerships is so overwhelming in health and social care policy that they are now a requirement rather than an option (Dowling et al. 2004, p. 309). The complexity and multidimensional nature of development problems necessitate a breadth and diversity of perspectives that cut across community sectors, and include external agencies. One community sector working alone is unlikely to be able to provide the breadth of expertise. From the community perspective, establishing partnerships usually leads to the acquisition of new resources. These may include financial support from external agencies, technical advice from consultants, and provision of opportunities to network regionally and nationally.

However, there is no one overarching reason why partnerships are established. Rather, the purpose, style, and nature of partnerships vary considerably, according

CASE EXAMPLE 9.1

The community garden

An inner-city neighbourhood centre had often thought about establishing a community vegetable garden. The suggestion had come from several residents who lacked the space where they lived to garden effectively, and who also wanted the social contact that such a project would provide. The first issue that the neighbourhood centre had to address was to find a suitable area for the garden. The centre's shop front location on a major road meant that it needed to form a partnership with an organisation that had land suitable for gardening and would agree to let the neighbourhood centre use it—the centre needed a 'host' organisation that had land and facilities to store gardening equipment. There were other needs, including financial support for equipment and expertise. Further, the neighbourhood centre in a nearby inner-city suburb had failed because of repeated vandalism of the garden, so some help with securing the garden was required.

Think about it

➤ What partnerships might be necessary if the neighbourhood centre is to find a location for the garden?
➤ What partnerships might help overcome the lack of resources?
➤ What partnerships might help overcome the security issues?

to community need and the nature of the task or the issue to be addressed. Some partnerships are short-term informal arrangements, while others are formalised in a non-legal partnership agreement. Occasionally, a legally binding contractual arrangement is entered into.

A proposal for a partnership may be prompted by community members who approach organisations to help them achieve a task. Other partnership proposals are instigated by external agencies when a partnership with a community is a prerequisite for making a funding application. Whatever the style of the partnership, there is always an acknowledgment that to solve a problem, or improve a situation, there will be a more effective result if the potential partners work together rather than separately (Bracht et al. 1999, p. 93).

The example of the neighbourhood community garden in case example 9.1 illustrates some of the reasons that lead to the formation of partnerships.

Practice tip 9.1

Partnerships building is sometimes called networking. For useful information on networking, go to the NSW Community Builders website: http://www.communitybuilders.nsw.gov.au/linking/networking

Key principles for effective partnership working

Wandersman et al. (2005, p. 292) describes bringing together diverse partners and running a successful coalition in health promotion as 'very hard work'. While there is advice about the ingredients for successful partnerships derived from experience, there is less information about how to deal with the very real tensions, dilemmas, and struggles about power-sharing that are common in partnership working (Balloch and Taylor 2001).

In practice, there is often an imperative for partnerships to achieve a goal or target quickly, so that the process of partnership building is neglected, or it is assumed that effective partnership functioning will occur given good will and hard work. On occasions, the disadvantages of partnering, such as the time involved in forming relationships, to negotiate different perspectives, and to build trust, may outweigh the advantages (Butterfoss et al. 1993, p. 322). In such cases, the imperative to partner may be based on ideological rather than pragmatic grounds (Dowling et al. 2004, p. 309).

Practice tip 9.2

Take time to check potential differences in perspectives early on rather than wait until problems arise.

Disagreements and friction in partnership working must be seen as inevitable, and may provide the fuel for partnership activity (Labonte 2005, p. 92). Power imbalances between communities, government agencies, and organisations always occur, and who is more, and who is less powerful in the partnership cannot be assumed without careful exploration. Therefore, the practice issues and skills involved in effective partnership working with communities require careful teasing out, identification, and development.

Three key elements underpinning the process of partnership working with communities are:

➤ achieving clarity regarding the purpose of the relationship and its goals and objectives (Roussos and Fawcett 2000, p. 383);
➤ building trusting relationships (Mohr and Spekman 1994, p. 138; Poland et al. 2005, p. 125); and
➤ achieving an understanding of collective efficacy (Johnson et al. 2003, p. 70).

Achieving clarity regarding the purpose of the partnership

Being clear about the purpose of the partnership involves discussing roles and the skills, experience, and resources that each will bring. In these negotiations, it is important that the stronger partners do not dominate the process to achieve their ends. Careful negotiation is necessary to ensure that unequal power relationships are managed (Poland et al. 2005, p. 125). Case example 9.2 illustrates how partners with less bargaining power may feel intimidated by a stronger partner.

Clarifying the purpose of the partnership is an ongoing process. Usually, as we shall see in the examples in this chapter, the initial purpose of the partnership may need adjustment over time as goals and objectives are achieved or change. It is quite common for partners to need to continually reassess the direction of partnerships, and this usually occurs through strategic planning. However, communities and organisations may be reluctant to do this when it may expose disagreements and bring unmanaged problems into the open.

There must be a continual focus on achieving the outputs required from the partnership. Often the reasons why the partnership was formed and the benefits it

CASE EXAMPLE 9.2

Purpose, partnership and power

A university wanted to partner with an Aboriginal community-controlled health service to apply for a research grant. The university provided funding for a much-needed staff position at the health service. Therefore the service felt obligated to partner with the University, even though the planned research was not in the service's priority area.

was to provide become unclear when those who established the partnership move on. Partnerships may persist for reasons other than those that were formally stated when they commenced. While there may be benefits in maintaining the partnership, it is important to acknowledge this and restate the new objectives and the expected outcomes.

In the following example, there are different perspectives on what a potential partnership may involve and what the benefits might be. It is almost always the case that there will be different perspectives on why a partnership should be formed.

CASE EXAMPLE 9.3

Partnerships for health promotion

A community health service in a city outer suburb established a partnership with the local school, the police service, and the youth accommodation agency to deliver a health promotion program about drug and alcohol misuse. From the perspective of the community health service, the purpose of the partnership was to engage with other agencies to strengthen the agency's strategic focus on addressing drug and alcohol misuse. From the perspective of the local school, this partnership was an opportunity to connect with an agency that, in the future, might run a range of health programs for them. The health promotion program proposed was not a police agency priority, and staff had very limited time to engage in community education programs. The youth accommodation agency had contact with a number of young adults who were most at risk of drug and alcohol abuse, but the service was not in agreement that this was the type of program that would be successful with their clients. They thought that their clients were often regarded as a 'captive audience' when it came to delivering health promotion programs, and youth shelter staff were very reluctant to insist on attendance.

Think about it

➤ What are the different perspectives on the goals of the partnership among the agencies?
➤ How might these be negotiated?
➤ What are the potential benefits of this partnership for each of the partners?

Trusting relationships

The extent to which communities and organisations share common interests is a major factor in considering how easy it is to establish trusting relationships to work together (Hord 1986, p. 26). Factors that assist trusting relationships include shared experiences, and a similar knowledge base and values. In addition, there are important contextual factors that affect the progress of partnerships, including resource issues and differences between partners' organisational culture. Mohr and Spekman (1994) found that higher levels of trust (the belief that one's word is reliable) between partners were associated with satisfaction with the partnership.

The factors that work against trusting relationships between partners attempting to collaborate to assist patient care across health and social services agencies in the UK have been identified as:

➤ differences in political views and therefore goals;
➤ fear of budgetary repercussions;
➤ differences between medical and social work cultures; and
➤ competing demands on overworked staff.

In the instances where collaboration did occur, it appeared that health and social work managers had similar goals, and they could articulate these clearly (Johnson et al. 2003 p. 80). In the community context, trusting relationships between community groups and individuals cannot be assumed. Often there are divisions between groups according to differences in socio-economic status, cultural background, or political views or interests. Some groups that are perceived to be divergent from the 'mainstream' culture may be excluded altogether (Bourke, 2001a, b).

To establish partnerships across different sections of the community, the skills involved are to identify the barriers to relationships, negotiate the differences between partners by establishing the common ground, and highlighting the benefits to each of the partners that will be gained from the partnership.

The following example illustrates the difficulties that may be encountered in establishing trusting relationships between organisations.

CASE EXAMPLE 9.4

Establishing trusting relationships

An Aboriginal community-controlled health service in a regional centre had struggled for many years to gain legitimacy among mainstream health providers. The service had a large geographic area to cover and provided a range of services beyond those traditionally classified as health services. Staff recruitment and retention was difficult, and although the service always wished to employ local Aboriginal or Torres Strait Islander people, there was a small pool of people to draw upon. The service had some different work practices from 'mainstream' health services, including a flexible appointment system and home visiting. When the staffing situation became acute, the service approached a community health service to assist with a recruitment and retention strategy. Although it wanted to help, the health service was uncomfortable with this as it didn't always support, or understand, the work practices in the Aboriginal service.

Think about it

➤ What are the relationship issues between these two agencies?

➤ What would be important factors in establishing trusting relationships?

➤ How do you think an effective partnership might be established?

Identifying mutual benefits

Both communities of place and of interest are usually well aware of their limitations in achieving their aspirations in economic and social development without the assistance of partners. Partnerships are built on an understanding that collaboration will bring benefits to the partners and that these benefits cannot be achieved by working alone. But in order to achieve these benefits, partners may have to put aside some of their priorities in order to join forces with others to achieve an overall objective (Butterfoss et al. 1993). Therefore, establishing partnerships inevitably means considering what each partner will gain and lose, and how the partnership can maximise mutual benefits. The benefits of partnering need to outweigh the disadvantages if the partnership is to be successful. The following example shows the complexities involved in weighing up the benefits of engaging in partnerships.

CASE EXAMPLE 9.5

Are there mutual benefits?

The regional health board wanted to increase its funding for primary health care. Funding could help establish a new community health centre in an outer metropolitan location and enable a new mental health program to operate. There was an announcement from a national mental health agency that funding would be available for community-based mental health programs, and the regional health board made enquiries. However, establishing a partnership with the national agency meant that all the programs provided would need to be approved by the agency, and would only be available for older adults. Board members then were in a dilemma as to whether they should accept funding and build a partnership.

Think about it?

➤ What success do you think the regional health board might have in negotiating with the national agency to meet some of their needs?
➤ What might be the difficulties in these negotiations?

The belief by partners in the concept of 'collective efficacy' needs to be present if responsibility is to be shared. That is, members of the partnership need to believe that the combined efforts of the group are not only necessary for group members to obtain the desired shared goal, but also that all members are capable of and willing to do their share of the work (Johnson et al. 2003 p. 70).

The following example illustrates the tensions involved in weighing up the benefits to communities in establishing a partnership with a property development company.

CASE EXAMPLE 9.6

A partnership to move the community house

The local government of an outer metropolitan area had received an offer from a development company to relocate the community house. There were plans for a new shopping centre in the area where the community house was currently located. The management committee had consulted with the community about the proposed relocation and received feedback that the proposal offered some benefits to the community. The major concern was whether or not the company would meet the community's requests regarding the new location for the community house.

Think about it

➤ What might be some of the benefits of a partnership with the development company for the community and the community house management committee?

➤ What might be some of the benefits for the development company?

➤ What might be the difficulties in ensuring both of the partners receive benefits from the partnership?

Types of partnerships

Partnerships within the community

In Chapter 2, the concepts of vertical and horizontal patterning of interactions (Warren 1978, p. 243) were used to understand the potential for collaborative activity, both within a community and between a community and individuals or groups that are external to it. While partnerships may, and usually do, involve both horizontal and vertical relationships, it is important to examine each separately.

Horizontal patterning is the structural and functional relationships of the community's various social units and subsystems to each other. Therefore, within-community partnerships involve the building of alliances of individuals and groups, both within and across sectors and interest groups, in order to achieve a common goal.

Within-sector partnerships

Within-sector partnerships are built around a social field (Wilkinson 1991 p. 36). In Chapter 2, a social field was described as the groups and organisations who come together to pursue their common objectives, such as the groups related to health, or the church organisations. Examples of within-sector partnerships are those between churches that share a common building, or within a health issues planning group that includes community health and hospital staff. These types of partnerships are likely to be strong when there is a clear purpose and evidence of mutual benefit from joining together to achieve a common goal.

Usually, these partnerships form spontaneously through interactions that arise in everyday life. They make sense because they are clearly fulfilling the social, business, spiritual, or recreational needs of community members, as was the case in the examples of the churches and the health planning group. Such partnerships need to be recognised because they demonstrate opportunities for existing relationships to be built upon. The following example is of strong within-sector partnerships that potentially may be utilised in community health or social care development.

CASE EXAMPLE 9.7

The annual football championship

The annual football championship in a regional centre brought together the clubs located throughout the region. The event, held over a long weekend, included social functions and an annual general meeting of the football association, as well as a football carnival. While, at first glance, the football championship may not be seen as relevant to community health or social care development, it demonstrates strong within-sector partnerships. Awareness of these partnerships provides opportunities to engage with significant numbers of people in the process of a community health or social care initiative.

Across-sector partnerships

In addition to within-sector partnerships, there are also partnerships that occur across community sectors. These across-sector partnerships are essential to community health and social care development because these are the ones that enable a community field to come together to solve problems, discuss issues, and work on new programs and initiatives. The concept of the community field, as a mechanism to bring people together to solve development problems of the entire community, was discussed in Chapter 2. Here is an example of across-sector partnerships that demonstrates the presence of a community field.

CASE EXAMPLE 9.8

The Winter Festival

The Winter Festival, sponsored by local government, was held annually in an inner city neighbourhood. It brought together local businesses, cultural groups, and community services. Events included bands, a street parade, school drama performances, and displays from local organisations. The festival had become a focal point in community life, partly because it had continued for many years and there was a history and traditions associated with it. The groups that worked together to hold the festival developed enduring relationships.

Think about it

➤ What might be some benefits for sectors in working together on the Winter Festival?

➤ What might be some challenges in maintaining working relationships over a long period of time?

Across-sector partnerships do not always happen spontaneously, because community interactions may persist around interest lines—such as the business sector or the health sector. When people are working hard together, it is sometimes easier to fall back on existing ties rather than engage in new relationships (Gittell and Vidal 1998, p. 175).

On occasions, the objective or goal of the partnership may not be community-driven, or 'ground up'. In Activity 9.1 (page 182), practitioners were obligated to run a communitywide 'across-sector' program in a community in order to meet an organisational objective. Therefore, the first step was the bringing together of across-sector partnerships that could help plan the initiative.

Finally, there are always competing priorities for people's time and commitment. Often, in small communities, there are numbers of partnerships already in place. Research participants in a study of community participation saw the following issues:

We see the same people all the time, the people who are on the hospital board are on the executive of the sporting clubs and they are also managing things for their

Activity 9.1

A crime prevention program

A crime prevention program required a partnership between schools, the business sector, and a neighbourhood watch program in order to access funding. In this urban neighbourhood, there were few informal links or networks between the education and business sectors, and the groups involved had never worked together before. The local development group was business-oriented and did not have an education sector representative. While the newly established neighbourhood watch program recognised the importance of the partnerships, its representatives thought the opportunity to obtain funding was too good to miss, and submitted the application with little consultation with the education or business sector. The application has been successful and it is your role as the community worker to help implement the program. What might be your first steps in implementing the program? How might consultation across sectors occur? What structures might be used to help the planning group?

church groups. People burn out and can't keep up the commitment but it is just how communities work and you get it everywhere. (Taylor 2004, p. 233)

Therefore new partnerships, even if they are to address an important issue, may be regarded with some trepidation.

The following example shows the ambivalence that people may have in forming across-sector partnerships when they involve new situations.

CASE EXAMPLE 9.9

Connecting with culturally and linguistically diverse communities

A community health centre in a regional city wanted to make its services more relevant to cultural and linguistically diverse communities. There were a number of groups representing diverse cultures who had little contact with the community health centre. The groups were unaware of the services provided, and were unsure as to whether they were eligible to attend. The staff at the centre had tried to make contact, but there were significant cultural and language differences. When a position became vacant at the centre, staff approached an experienced community health nurse, recently arrived from Ethiopia, was asked to apply. Although there were problems with recognition of qualifications, these were worked through. The new staff member suggested numerous changes to the programs and staff practices for the different groups to feel comfortable to attend the centre. While willing to consider the changes, the centre was unconvinced that the time and resources involved could be justified. They argued that there were only a few families from each cultural group and it could be the role of the community health nurse to act as the go-between rather than change programs and practices.

Think about it

➤ Why was the community health centre interested in forming partnerships with culturally and linguistically diverse groups in the community?

➤ Why was the health centre ambivalent about the benefits of the partnership?

➤ Why might the health centre be reluctant to make changes to programs and practices?

➤ Would it be appropriate for the community health nurse to be the go-between?

Partnerships with those external to the community

Vertical patterning is the relationship between a community's social units and systems outside it (Martinez-Brawley 2000, pp. 71–84). External partnerships are those that involve building relationships between community groups and external government agencies, experts, and development organisations. Most community health and social care development involves partnerships of this nature because of the complexity of problems to be addressed. Communities may not have all the resources that are required to undertake development, and partnerships may assist in obtaining these resources. Activity 9.2 demonstrates this.

'Bridging social capital' is a term that can be used to describe these vertical ties that assist development through forming bridges between communities and resource agencies. Putnam distinguished between two types of social capital. The first, bonding social capital, brings people closer together who already know each other. The second, bridging social capital, brings people together who do not know each other (Gittell and Vital 1998, p. 175).

Activity 9.2

Partnerships to access funding

A community worker was aware of funding being made available for parenting programs in rural and remote locations if communities could join together across regional areas. The regional development organisation sponsored the application and provided the resources for community representatives to meet together to discuss it. As the community worker involved, your task is to plan for and convene the meeting of the community representatives. What topics should be on the agenda at the first meeting?

In community health and social care development, a balance of horizontal and vertical ties, and bridging and bonding capital is necessary. This will ensure the participation both of those who have local roots and across-sector ties within the community and those people outside the community who can bring in new information and expertise. These partnerships ensure that expertise brought to the community is imbued with local knowledge. It is then more likely that development will be locally owned, relevant, and sustainable.

Negotiating the balance of external and internal partnerships demands a sound understanding of the existing community networks and an ability to make linkages between existing networks and external resources. Achieving this balance of relationships is complex, as the following example illustrates.

CASE EXAMPLE 9.10

The Domestic Violence Coalition

Most key service providers in a regional city regarded the problem of violence towards older people as a serious one. In order to address this, the aged care sector, a women's shelter, the police agency, and the income security agency had established a community-based action group. The objective was to increase community awareness of the problem, provide more integrated service delivery for those affected, and to advocate for more effective policy to address the issue. The organisations involved had different perspectives on the problem and different responsibilities, and most were extremely busy.

It was difficult to get community groups involved, as there was a lack of awareness that there was a problem. Due to this, the organisations involved began to look for external support, and engaged with state and national networks to address the issues. Connections between the action group and the regional community became tenuous.

Think about it

➤ What are the within-community partnerships that make up the action group?
➤ What are the partnerships involved that are external to the community?
➤ What are some of the issues in balancing the within-community partnerships with the external partnerships?

Partnership development

The development of partnerships can be divided into three phases: the joining phase, during which the partners are recruited and the purpose of the partnership is clarified; the working phase, during which partnerships become productive; and the moving-on phase, when the outcomes have been achieved. Research on partnerships and coalitions has identified particular skills needed in order to achieve each of these phases of partnership development effectively (Butterfoss et al. 1993, p. 319).

The formation phase

In facilitating the formation of partnerships, the skills involved are:

➤ clarifying and negotiating the exchange of resources between partners—who brings what to the partnership;
➤ identifying to potential partners how the benefits from the partnerships outweigh the disadvantages; and
➤ the ability to draw together sufficient organisations or communities to enable the partnership to realise the benefits.

Overall, it is the clarity of the objective of the partnership, and whether or not there will be benefits for the potential partners that influences becoming a member. The setting for the following activity is a situation in which a partnership might realise benefits if each of the four regions would agree to participate.

Activity 9.3

Deciding whether or not to form a partnership

Human service delivery was being reorganised and there was an opportunity for four existing regions to join together to coordinate their services, gain increased resources, and have one overall governance arrangement. Three regions were interested, but the fourth, the region that covered rural and remote areas, was reluctant. Because its population was smaller than the other regions and the costs of service delivery were higher, this region thought that it might not receive the resources it required. If you were to be the facilitator to help regions decide whether or not to amalgamate, what steps would you take in this process? What issues need to be considered?

Where there is a history of cooperation, a new partnership proposal may be readily accepted because partners already know each other's way of working and there are trusting relationships. If the partnership is between communities and organisations that have not previously worked together, then relationship building may take time, and requires a conciliatory rather than a directive approach.

Activity 9.4

Coordinating response to a traumatic event

Human and health services in an outer-urban neighbourhood needed to coordinate efforts to respond to a serious school bus crash. Most of the service delivery to the neighbourhood was on an outreach basis and there were few working partnerships and limited experience in working together.

Think about it

➤ What are the issues involved in establishing partnerships in the context of this traumatic event?

➤ How might some of these issues be managed?

Achieving these working relationships is difficult when timeframes are short, as is likely, for example, in the case of submitting a grant application for a project involving several partners. In such a situation, partnership formation may be abbreviated and partners may sign up to the partnership on the basis that 'the details can be sorted out later'. To establish effective partnerships in this context requires skilled leadership and realistic expectations of what can be achieved within a short timeframe.

It is also difficult to achieve partnerships in situations that demand an immediate response if there are few prior working relationships. Activity 9.4 demonstrates this point.

Formalised partnership agreements

Most authors agree that the objectives, roles, and responsibilities of the partnership should be negotiated and formalised in a written partnership agreement, and that this supports the maintenance of the partnership (Butterfoss et al. 1993, p. 321). Examples of written agreements include mission statements, memoranda of understanding, and letters of agreement. Often, the first meeting of the partners involves deciding on the objectives, roles and responsibilities of the partnership, noting these in the minutes, and circulating them to partners.

Partnership agreements are a way of making clear to all parties the purposes, roles, and responsibilities involved, and they assist in evaluating the effectiveness of the partnership as it continues. The process of negotiating the agreement is of value in itself as it often introduces opportunities to discuss aspects that are not clear, or issues that had not been thought of.

The following checklist identifies the components that may be relevant for a partnership agreement.

Practice tip 9.3

Checklist for a partnership agreement:

- ➤ The contact details of those organisations/communities who constitute partnership
- ➤ The purpose of the partnership and the expected outcomes
- ➤ The roles and responsibilities of each of the partners
- ➤ The lead agency or community
- ➤ The resources available
- ➤ The timeframe for the partnership
- ➤ How the partnership will be evaluated.

Activity 9.5

Writing a partnership agreement

The neighbourhood centre referred to in Case example 9.1 had been able to gain access to a small amount of land at the local primary school on which to establish the community garden. The local school was keen for its students to participate in gardening activities. Your task is to write an agreement that will help ensure that the partnership is effective in enabling the community garden to operate well.

Informal partnerships

The informal working partnerships between community sectors and regions are important to acknowledge. While there may be no formal partnership agreement, there may be ongoing mutually beneficial working relationships that have evolved to undertake community projects. Trying to formalise these relationships may cost time and energy, and may not result in increased effectiveness. An observation by a research participant illustrates some problems of trying to formalise what has been an informal arrangement between community organisations.

Activity 9.6

Informality or a written agreement?

Three communities who had been affected by serious flooding agreed to work together to put on a concert to raise funds for those who had been affected by the event. All the communities had worked together before and had existing communication systems, ways of sharing resources, and identified leaders. There was a view that a written partnership agreement would be inappropriate, given that there were ongoing relationships.

Think about it

➤ Should the objectives and roles and responsibilities of the partnership be clarified in this situation?
➤ Would a written partnership agreement be necessary?

The health service is trying to encourage a partnership between all the agencies in the region but I consider the way the structure is set up it is discouraging this. There is too much time spent on paper work and memorandums and the like. Because of the amount of bureaucracy and red tape it is just too much for many of the local people. (Taylor 2004, p. 152)

Just as important are the external connections with organisations, consultants, and technical advisers who provide resources and support. Formalising these relationships through written partnership agreements would be inappropriate. The value of the connections is that they can be activated on a 'needs basis' and there is no long-term commitment.

The working phase

The working phase of the partnership can be considered from two perspectives: how well partners work together in addressing their joint aims; and whether or not the outcomes of the partnership are achieved. To date, studies on partnerships have focused heavily on process issues, and success in achieving outcomes is given much less emphasis (Dowling et al. 2004, p. 309).

Practice tip 9.4

Ensure that there are quantifiable indicators of specific service delivery outcomes that could not be achieved without the partnership.

While it is necessary to add to the evidence about the impacts on clients or end users of partnerships, the research on process issues is useful, especially that concerning the factors contributing to successful health promotion coalitions (Ansari et al. 2001; Butterfoss et al. 1996; Granner and Sharpe 2004). From the literature, three areas are identified as important in forming successful partnerships:

➤ communication (Mohr and Spekman 1994);
➤ maintaining motivation (Butterfoss et al. 1996); and
➤ the organisational and policy context (Poland et al. 2005).

Communication

Communication underlies the effectiveness of partnership functioning, and in fact partnerships happen through communication. Strategies that support high-quality communication and information flow build a sense of commitment to the partnership (Mohr and Spekman 1994, p. 148). Effective communication between partners helps establish a common purpose and focus, increases trust, and enables resource sharing (Butterfoss et al. 1996, p. 324).

However, effective communication is hard to achieve when there are competing demands on people's time and there are different views to be listened to and incorporated into plans. Therefore, it is important for all partners to understand that communication underpins partnerships and may be facilitated through face-to-face interactions. Frequent meetings may help, and there are technical aids such as video-conferencing facilities. On the other hand, the frequency of meetings must be carefully determined, as expectations to attend too many meetings may impose on partners' goodwill.

Communication should involve real dialogue that explores all the perspectives on the task and the process of achieving the task (Labonte 2005, p. 92). Managing unequal power relationships is necessary to ensure this dialogue occurs. Unequal power relationships may also affect the flow of information, with important information being shared only with powerful or high-performing partners. If up-to-date information is not available equally to all partners, then partners may not be able to complete their tasks effectively (Mohr and Spekman 1994, p. 139).

The partnership environment

The environments in which partnerships operate also affect their success. A supportive policy environment will assist in overcoming systemic barriers to collaboration. For instance, Poland and others' (2005) study of partnerships between communities and hospitals showed that hospital organisational policies, structures, and culture did not always support the ways in which communities wished to work. While hospitals stated that they supported partnerships with communities, the policy and fiscal environment demanded that hospitals should maintain control, and this did not contribute to effective involvement.

In some marginalised communities, patterns of racial discrimination and a low resource base may inhibit effective partnerships. The commitment of resources by these communities may be difficult even if the partnership is to result in a much needed service or activity. There are always competing demands, and communities will engage in those partnerships that will realise the greatest benefit (Fawcett et al. 1995, p 693).

Maintaining motivation

The effort that communities and organisations put into partnerships must be continually rewarded in order for the partnership to continue. Rewards come from both task achievement and the partnership process. If the objective of the partnership is complex or involves change in attitudes and behaviours, then the momentum required to sustain partnerships may come from one or more 'champions on the ground' (Poland et al. 2005, p. 127).

If task achievement is straightforward and results in new services or activities that clearly benefit the community, then motivation may be more easily maintained. Motivation may be strengthened by community members' awareness that they are fulfilling their duty to community through working together on community projects (Butterfoss et al.1996; Taylor et al. 2005). The primary impetus for the formation of a partnership may contribute to its ability to be maintained. For instance, if partnerships are initiated primarily to secure funding and it is the fundholder who receives most of the benefits, then partnerships may falter. However, if partnerships are initiated by communities to gain needed technical expertise, and government agencies are obtaining experience through the process, then motivation may be sustained.

Activity 9.7

The partnership working phase

A formal partnership between four diverse communities was entered into to obtain funding for a suicide prevention program. One of the communities did much of the work to bring the partnership together, made the funding application, and became the fundholder. Now that the funds have been received and the project has commenced, the lead community is struggling to maintain the involvement of the other communities.

Think about it

➤ What factors might assist in getting involvement from all four communities in the suicide prevention project?

Moving on

The ending phase of a partnership is when the objectives have been achieved. It is important that partners acknowledge this phase and plan for it effectively. Both ensuring closure and celebrating achievements are important aspects of completing partnerships.

Ensuring closure

The length of the partnership is not necessarily an indicator of partnership effectiveness. Some partnerships continue on long after the objectives have been achieved, and this can be for several reasons. First, it may be satisfying to partners to maintain their close working relationships, and if this is not hindering the development of new projects, then this is appropriate. However, often energy may need to be directed to building new partnerships with new goals and objectives. Usually it is the familiar partnership that will be preferred.

Generally partners can see when the task has been achieved or when it is clear that the partnership is no longer functional. The brevity of some partnerships may reflect that there has been a clear understanding of the purpose and intent of the partnership. On the other hand, it may be that the partnership is inappropriate, and it is better to end it sooner rather than later. Carefully terminating an unsatisfactory partnership may be an appropriate resolution. Ending partnerships requires sensitive management so that partners may reflect on what they have achieved and the strengths and limitations of the partnership have been acknowledged. If this is not the case, then unresolved issues may interfere with effective relationships in the future (Bringle and Hatcher 2002, p. 511).

Activity 9.8

Ending partnerships

A university campus partnered with three urban neighbourhoods to achieve funding for an exercise program for primary school students. The partnership continued for six months with clear goals and objectives, and cooperative working relationships. Approximately 200 children participated in the programs, two neighbourhoods are continuing to run the programs although the funding has ceased, and several primary schools are incorporating the programs into their activities.

Think about it

➤ What would be important in ensuring appropriate closure for this partnership?

➤ What would be some of the ways that the achievements of the partnership could be celebrated?

Celebrating achievements

One of the important aspects in terminating partnerships is to celebrate the achievements in an appropriate manner. If a new service has been established or resources acquired, then an 'open day' is one way for communities and their partners to show off their accomplishments. Communicating the outcomes of the partnership in community newsletters or in the media is also effective. It is important that those who have been involved in working in partnership have a chance to reflect on the partnership's strengths. Having some type of formal event makes this easier.

SUMMARY

Community partnerships involve sectors, agencies, technical advisers, and practitioners, working together to achieve mutually agreed goals. Both the processes involved in the working relationships are important as well as the outcomes. Most evaluation of partnerships has focused on the nature of the working relationships rather than the outcomes, and a concentration on the latter is essential. There are three key components of effective partnerships: achieving clarity regarding the purpose of the relationship; building trusting relationships; and achieving a shared understanding of collective efficacy.

Within-community partnerships are described as horizontal, and involve both across-sector and within-sector relationships. Those partnerships that bring in expertise from outside the community are external or vertical partnerships. The skill involved is balancing the horizontal with vertical partnerships to ensure that local communities can contribute knowledge that informs the contribution of external agencies.

The development of partnerships can be divided into three phases: the joining phase, during which the partners are recruited and the purpose of the partnership is clarified; the working phase, during which partnerships become productive; and the moving-on phase, when the outcomes have been achieved. Each of these phases requires particular skills to assist partnerships function effectively, maintain motivation, be sustainable in order to achieve the partnership objectives, and achieve satisfactory closure when it is time to move on.

USEFUL WEBSITES

Resources for partnership development

The URP Toolbox: https://www3.secure.griffith.edu.au/03/toolbox

The Australian Government Community website—information about community
partnerships:

http://www.community.gov.au/Internet/MFMC/Community.nsf/pages/section?open
document&Section=Community%20Partnership

The NSW Government Community Builders: http://www.communitybuilders.nsw.
gov.au

Community Development Toolkit, University of Louisiana: http://ctb.ku.edu

Mentoring social enterprises

Grassroots Networking Foundation promoting civil and democratic communities:
http://www.grassroots.org.au

Social Ventures Partnerships: http://www.socialventures.com.au/home.asp

CHAPTER 10

Community Leadership

Introduction

This chapter on community leadership builds on the information presented in the previous chapters about partnerships and decision-making. In this chapter, we introduce the relational approach to leadership and apply this to community leadership. Several issues that are common to achieving sustainable leadership in communities of place and of interest are examined, and three key elements of community leadership are presented: creating a common purpose; bringing people together; and balancing task and group processes. The chapter concludes with some exercises that may assist in community leadership development.

What is community leadership?

Community leadership involves complex, often challenging, and non-linear processes. There is often no clear cause-and-effect relationship between leadership and community project outcomes. In our rational systems-oriented paradigm, we tend to visualise a process as something that can be represented by a flow chart with clear relationships between each aspect. But it is not like this with community leadership. The process involves people interacting, having their say, disagreeing, forming coalitions, and eventually out of this comes some direction and a common interest. Leadership is a process of change in which it may be difficult to clearly identify what impact a leader has had or even who the leader is. The following observation by a community leader illustrates how this person sees community leadership.

> We had to get some donations and get people to use the new service we had established. Most of us belong to church; we stand around and chat and you can do a great deal of lobbying for our projects after church. Most of us also belong to sporting organisations. You can do a great deal of good there but you have to get off your bike and do something. It is up to community leaders to work through the community. (Taylor, 2004, p. 57)

The approach to community leadership used in this chapter is the relational approach, chosen because of its focus on process, interactions, and influence relationships (Rost 1993). The notion of relational leadership sits comfortably with the community interaction theory approach to understanding community functioning that was presented in Chapter 2.

The relational approach to community leadership

Leadership, according to Rost (1993, p. 99), involves 'an influence relationship among leaders and collaborators who intend real changes that reflect their mutual purposes'. Influence relationships emerge from a culture of trust, and involve the unified action of leaders and followers. It is not about what is 'done' to followers by leaders, but rather it is a process of mutual influence (Pigg 1999, p. 200). Relational leadership then is more about interactions and the processes of influence between leaders and their constituents rather than the views of leadership that rest on formal positions, authority, skill sets, and leaders' behaviours.

Applying this understanding to community leadership, it is clear that it involves building relationships to bring people together to work towards a common purpose in a community of place or of interest. The common purpose is always related to community benefit. It could be to obtain ideas about how to solve a community issue, plan for a new service, or lobby for a desired change. This relational view of community leadership has 'influence' relationships between leaders and their constituents or collaborators at the heart of the processes.

Understanding leadership in communities differs from understanding organisational leadership. Community leaders operate in the community rather than in an organisation, and they cannot rely on formal authority or the power derived from positions to get things done. 'Instead, they must rely on networks and influence, with relationships developed through extensive interactions with community residents usually representing many different points of view or interests' (Pigg 1999, p. 196, quoting O'Brien and Hassinger, 1992).

In contrast, organisational leadership involves managing staff to achieve organisational goals. Leadership then becomes an overarching competency relevant to most aspects of the management function. The ability to influence comes primarily from the leader's position in the organisational structure, and the manager enacts leadership because of the position he or she holds in the organisation (Hartley 1996).

Four elements of relational leadership

Rost's (1993, pp. 99–100) definition of relational leadership involves four key elements:

➤ the leadership relationship is based in multi-directional influence;

➤ followers are active in the relationship and there may be more than one leader;

➤ leaders and their constituents intend, but do not necessarily produce, real changes; and

➤ the changes that the leaders and their collaborators intend reflect their mutual purposes.

This example illustrates these four elements.

CASE EXAMPLE 10.1

Community leadership in a community of interest

The Iraqi community wanted to address the growing problem of obtaining affordable housing for community members. Increasing costs of rental and home ownership in the town were the reasons usually given for the problem. Community members had discussed the housing issues for several years, and the situation came to a head when several newly arrived families could not find housing. Several women who were related to the families concerned decided to tackle the issue. They approached their religious leaders, who gave their support and made contact with a national housing society that had information about developing low-cost housing options. Women visited the families they knew who might understand the problem and help work to address it. Using resources from the community and external sources, community leaders organised a well-attended meeting, and a working group was formed with the idea of starting a housing cooperative. From the meeting, it was clear that starting a housing cooperative would be a longer-term plan, but there were other suggestions that could help alleviate the immediate housing situation.

Think about it

➤ How is leadership demonstrated through this example?
➤ Who are the leaders?
➤ How do the leaders influence others?
➤ What were the changes that the leaders intended?
➤ Were these changes achieved?

In this scenario, some community members influenced others to join forces to tackle a community problem. The influence relationships were multi-dimensional and came about because of existing networks. Some community members had the commitment, the time and the energy to encourage others to work together to benefit the community.

In this case, the leaders had existing relationships that they could call on. They didn't have to start from scratch, making themselves known to people, discussing what they would like to do for the community, and building trusting relationships. However, leadership can evolve without these connections—it just takes longer. Building relationships of trust where there are no existing connections usually works best if the leader can be 'introduced' to the community and a place can be

CASE EXAMPLE 10.2

Joining together to lobby local government

Local government in a regional centre on the coast proposed to develop the foreshore by putting in a new road close to the beach. This proposal meant that the children's playground and lawn area would be on the other side of the road, and children would need to cross the road to access the beach. Several community leaders were opposed to the proposal because of this, and encouraged residents to form a community action group. The community action group held meetings, lobbied the local government, and distributed flyers. Although the group was unsuccessful in halting the development proposal, it had brought people together around a common issue, and the group continued to advocate on other development issues.

found for that person within existing networks. This 'easing in process' typifies community relational leadership. In contrast, organisational leaders can take up a leadership role because of a formal position they hold in an organisation. Leadership is an assumed status that comes with a position.

Relational leadership is about the leadership process and creating a common purpose or intent just as much as it is about the achievement of a specific goal. This means that leadership may persist even if the tasks that leaders and their constituents had in mind were not achieved. If community members know that they are working towards a common purpose, and the purpose is to benefit the community, then whether or not the specific task is achieved may not affect leadership (Pigg 1999, p. 202). This is a really important point, and may explain why some communities continue to work on tasks that from the outside seem impossible to achieve. Having a joint interest in community development is what underpins community leadership and keeps it going. Case example 10.2 illustrates this point.

Influence relationships

Effective influence relationships may at various times be authoritative, affiliative, democratic, pacesetting, and coaching (Goleman 1998). For example, in leading a community planning session, there will be expectations of what type of product will be produced, and the leader will take an authoritative role to see that this is achieved. However, there will be opportunities to get community members involved by taking advice from them and reinforcing appropriate suggestions that are made—these are affiliative and coaching relationships. Whatever the style of leadership, there must always be some level of agreement between leaders and community members about what the common purpose is, and this is negotiated without formal authority to enforce the leaders' view. Coercion may be involved initially to encourage people to get involved, but unless there are effective relationships between leaders and constituents, it is unlikely that people will continue to be involved. Overall, there is a reliance on relationships and goodwill between leaders and community members rather than coercion.

People who can establish and maintain influence relationships are likely to have sound communication skills, and they are likely to be influential and persuasive. They may use five important communication skills—enabling, enlisting, entrusting, engaging, and envisioning—to get their views across. What is very important to note is that, although possessing these skills may facilitate leadership, it is a two-way process, and community members may react differently to the leader's intentions and communication style (Ponce 1995, p. 68). Underlying effective communication skills are trusting relationships.

Practice tip 10.1

While good communication is important, leadership is more than communication. It is about relationships.

Another feature of influence relationships is that they are inherently unequal because the influence patterns are unequal. Some people have more ability to convey their views and understand those of others, and can give stronger form and direction to the relationship. They can influence others to become involved and share their vision with them.

Activity 10.1

Identifying influence relationships

Choose a community of place or community of interest that you are familiar with. If you wanted to get the community involved in a health development or social care community project, who would you approach? Why would you approach that person? What influence does that person have with community members?

Shared leadership

Leadership is a multi-directional process between leaders and their constituents. It can be distributed throughout a community. It can involve anybody, not only those who hold formal positions in the public sphere (Kirk and Shutte 2004, p. 236). Practitioners, religious leaders, young people, volunteers, business people, and government personal can all be leaders if they can establish influence relationships with community members. There is a difference in this approach from the Alinsky model of community organising, which maintains a distinction between public sphere leaders called organisers and the private sphere community leaders. In Alinsky's model, the impetus for leadership is external, and results in empowerment of local people. In this model, leadership evolves through communitywide relationships (Stall and Stoecker 1998, p. 743).

In communities of place, community leadership may be undertaken by those who do not hold a position of authority in an organisation, but who are active and have connections across the community. Sorenson and Epps (1996,

p. 118), in research identifying community leaders in four country towns in Central Queensland, found that relatively few key leaders occupied a position of authority. Rather, the most effective leaders were people who were active across the community, had links externally, and had a communitywide vision.

This is not to say that people who hold formal roles in health and human services cannot be community leaders. But it is the nature of their relationships with others rather than their formal position that will determine what leadership roles they will play. For example, the community health worker may wish to implement an innovative preventative health program at the neighbourhood centre. But the worker has only recently moved to the area and is not well linked to community networks. It would be difficult to use the position alone to gain sufficient support for the program. The community worker will 'ask around' to find community members who are likely to benefit from the program and who have networks that the community worker can become part of.

The following activity demonstrates how leadership in tackling a community problem may be shared between community leaders and external resource people.

CASE EXAMPLE 10.3

Sharing leadership to tackle a difficult issue

A culturally and linguistically diverse (CALD) community was struggling to address the problem of domestic violence. While everybody knew there was a problem, it was rarely spoken about. From a religious perspective, violence toward women and children was unacceptable, and yet those who were experiencing the problem kept it hidden. Some community members thought that it might be possible to provide some education programs in the community. These community leaders took up the issue with a community worker who was known and trusted by the community. They suggested that a program would be led by the community worker, and that the local leaders would encourage people to attend.

Think about it

➤ Why did community people suggest the community worker run the domestic violence program?
➤ Why did the community leaders suggest they could encourage attendance?

Gender and community leadership

Gender may be a factor in establishing influence relationships to bring people together around a common purpose. Stall and Stoecker (1998, p. 774) note that community organising typically begins with the expanded private sphere of the neighbourhood. It is in this space that women may have extensive relationships and may connect strongly around local issues. There are many examples of a women-centred model of community organising in establishing women's refuges, women's health centres, and rape crisis services in Australia and internationally.

Women's organising may be facilitated by the relationships that leaders have with local networks that are built through everyday activities. Because of these connections, women may know what is going on in the community and be able to communicate this information. In the following case example, a research participant reflects on her volunteering role.

CASE EXAMPLE 10.4

Community women's networks

Source: Taylor, 2004, p. 189

As community women, we used to be involved in the hospital board as community representatives. This is important because we know what is going on. We could go to a board meeting where there are five or six men and possibly three women, and the men didn't have any idea about some of the things that were happening in the community. They were just not at the places we would go to. We would visit all the elderly people with 'meals on wheels', so we knew their problems. We know about the young ones and how they have to leave town for employment. Women are out in the community all the time volunteering. We know that men have to have 9–5 jobs, and we as women didn't have that opportunity.

The emergence of leadership in some community settings may be facilitated when there are close relationships between leaders and their constituents. In the example above, some of the older women in the community felt that through their networks they had a sound knowledge of the community issues. Using Robnett's (1996) term, these women could be described as 'centre-women'. Centre-women can link people across several networks and may be able to transform social networks into action groups when there are problems and issues. The other point is that women may be able to translate the negotiation skills that are learnt in their families into the public sphere.

CASE EXAMPLE 10.5

Using women's networks in a family planning initiative

Source: Shiffman 2002, p. 1199

A government family planning initiative in Indonesia drew on local women's groups as a starting point in providing family planning education. This starting point was chosen because the groups were embedded in local communities, but they were also networked across regions. They had an active membership interested in improving women's and children's health and wellbeing.

Some challenges of community leadership

The challenges involved in achieving effective community leadership are apparent in at least two areas: first, ensuring that there is a spread of leadership throughout the community; and second, ensuring sustainability and preventing burnout.

A spread of leadership

In many small communities, a handful of local leaders may contribute heavily to the process of community action (Israel and Beaulieu 1990, p. 188). Research in rural Australian communities finds that the same few people may put up their hands and get involved in several leadership positions in the community. A research participant explains this.

> We see the same people all the time as leaders, the people who are on the hospital board are on the executive of the sporting clubs, and they are also managing things for their church groups. It is just different groups of people and you get it everywhere. There are people who are happy to make decisions and take responsibility for things, then there will be another group who get involved at work, then there is a group that doesn't want to do anything. (Research participant, Taylor 2004)

Leaders who emerge may not necessarily be well linked to different groups, sectors or social fields. In small communities, whether of place or of interest, having someone to take on leadership roles is better than having no-one at all, even if that person is not seen as well linked.

Practice tip 10.2

Committed community members with energy and enthusiasm for community development are a very important resource in small communities, and it is important to work with this resource.

Eyre and Gauld (2003, p. 195) assessed community participation in developing a health service in rural New Zealand, and found that leadership largely emerged through a process of self-selection, commitment to volunteer work, and community service. Leaders emerged from groups and sectors that were similar in levels of affluence and age, but they did not represent marginalised groups. However, they were able to develop a highly regarded and well-used community health trust.

Making leadership sustainable

Another problem in a community with a limited number of potential leaders is that people may become overcommitted, or wear 'too many hats', and burn out. People are frequently unaware that this is occurring, and the following reflection by a research participant illustrates this.

> The consequences for me [of establishing a new service] were once we had finished and we had our doctors in place and things were going really well I fell down a big hole. Now I am really tired. Fortunately with my job change now I decided to resign from the board for a while and I am enjoying the break. It was a sense of release to resign and have a breather now, but 'burnout' was probably the right word. I didn't think of that at the time, looking back. (Taylor 2004, p. 220)

While community leaders may be effective, have appropriate skills, and be able to motivate community members to join with them, they may do this at a personal cost. Unless there is appropriate mentoring for leaders to acknowledge when they may need to withdraw and have a break, the situation may escalate.

The final section of this chapter provides some exercises to assist communities obtain a spread of leadership, run leadership training events, and put in place safeguards against burnout.

Community leadership skills

The skills involved in relational leadership in health and social care development are generic. They can be applied both in communities of place and of interest, and in all kinds of community development. 'Community leadership may involve the use of power to influence decisions concerning local programs, may guide the activities of other participants, or may include "rolling up the sleeves" and pitching in to get the job done' (Israel and Beaulieu 1990, p. 186). It is not so much the type of activity that leaders undertake that is important, it is the purpose of the activity. There are three key areas in which leadership is crucial in health and social care development. These are:

➤ being able to generate a common purpose or area of interest around which activity occurs;
➤ bringing different groups in a community together to build the community field; and
➤ balancing task achievement with group maintenance functions.

Creating a common purpose

One of the essential skills in community leadership is the ability to bring people together around a common purpose. Leaders rely on their relationships with community members to engage with them and discuss what needs to be done and how people think it can be done.

However, if there is to be a shared purpose, then leaders need to be able to do more than collect different perspectives. They also need to be able to integrate different views into a shared view. This is often the most important and difficult aspect of the leadership process. The concept of transformational leadership (Bass 1999) is useful in understanding more about how to develop a common purpose.

Transformational leadership

Transformational leadership refers to moving followers or constituents beyond immediate self-interest to consider a greater good that will result from sharing a common interest. It is about inspiring change and growth. Certain characteristics assist this process, including an ability to form relationships, charisma, capacity to portray a desirable future, intellectual stimulation, and identifying how individual needs can be met through the process (Bass 1999).

Although the concept of transformational leadership has been developed in relation to organisational leadership, it has relevance to community leadership.

Transformational community leaders will engender loyalty, commitment, involvement, and performance of followers if they are able to identify a community interest that will encompass most individual interests. Then people will feel that their interests can be met and they will be willing to get involved.

Research has identified some important aspects of transformational leadership. Transformational leaders can be directive or participative, authoritarian, or democratic, and they usually incorporate several leadership styles. Studies have suggested that women may be more transformational in their leadership than men (Bass et al. 1996), and attributes correlated with transformational leadership, such as facilitating and nurturing, are qualities traditionally associated with women's roles in our society (Ross and Offerman 1997, p. 1084). Again, gender may play a role in leadership styles.

Aligning personal interests with community interests

A critical factor related to health and social care development is to create a common interest that will benefit the whole community rather than just a few. To do this, community leaders will develop strategies so that personal interests can be meshed with community interests, or at least ensure that there is some agreement.

In some cases, personal interests and community interests go hand in hand, and there is a natural synergy between them. For example, there is increasing evidence that participation in community improvement projects is motivated, in part, by a wanting to gain a sense of community connectedness resulting from joint action. Therefore, involvement in the development project helps both the individual and the community. Here is an example of how a new arrival to a community gained a sense of belonging through membership of a group helping to establish health facilities.

> I am new to this community and one of my motivations for contributing is maintaining my own place in the community to some extent but it has a community benefit. We really need to improve our aged care facilities and you never know I may need them some day! (Taylor 2004, p. 128)

On the other hand, there are situations where it is very difficult to align individual interests with a common purpose. Case example 10.6 illustrates this.

Leadership to bring private and community interests together in this situation involved ensuring that people's concerns about traffic and property prices were appropriately dealt with. Community leaders also worked on building relationships between community members who supported the child care centre and those who didn't, to share information about the need for child care. There was also an opportunity to focus on some of the potential benefits of having a centre in the neighbourhood that had been overlooked.

CASE EXAMPLE 10.6

Should the neighbourhood centre sponsor a child care centre?

A neighbourhood in an inner city was divided over whether or not a child care centre should be built in the area. For the neighbourhood centre, which was to be the sponsor of the project, it was an opportunity to provide much-needed and affordable child care places. However, in obtaining community views, the neighbourhood centre found most people were against the proposal. They were afraid that property prices might deteriorate, traffic might be increased when parents dropped off and picked up their children, and parking might become more of a problem.

Activity 10.2

Aligning individual and community interests

In Case example 10.6, about building the child care centre, some of the private interests that would motivate community members to oppose and support building the child care centre have been identified. What are other private interests that might be operating? What are some of the community benefits of having the child care centre in the area that could be highlighted?

Developing the community field

Central to all aspects of community leadership in health and social care development is the ability to bring different community sectors and interest groups together for community development. This is known as building the community field. The community field, as discussed in Chapter 2, 'involves a process of inter-related actions through which residents express their common interest in the local society' (Wilkinson 1991, p. 2).

The community field is built around general community interests rather than those that are related to a specific sector or interest group. Therefore, developing the community field involves leadership that assists community residents to create, maintain, and enhance generalised community structures and interactions. For example, the neighbourhood centre's plan to sponsor a child care centre (Case example 10.6) involved bringing together the planning sector, residents' groups, and local government. Networks that are established because of the child care centre discussions can be used again for different issues.

Community attachment

Research in rural communities has shown that where there are strong emotional and sentimental attachments to the social and natural environments where people live, there may also be strong motivations to develop and sustain them (Wilkinson 1991, p. 69). Because of these attachments, the community field may emerge strongly, especially when the wellbeing of the community is threatened (Tilley 1973). Then it may be easier to bring people together.

It may also be easier to bring people together if the initiator can be seen to be part of the local community and acting on the community's behalf. Some research has also shown that in rural communities, attachment to the local community is a necessary prerequisite for leaders to become involved in the process of mobilising for social change.

However, the relationship between community attachment and leadership is complex (O'Brien and Hassinger 1992, p. 532). Leaders who are strongly attached to their community and who have lived there a long time may have strong ties, but also have restricted access to external information networks (Granovetter 1973). On the other hand, leaders who are new to the community may not be 'attached',

CASE EXAMPLE 10.7

Including minority groups

Source: Campbell and McLean 2002, pp. 643–57

In a deprived, multi-ethnic area of a town in southern England, African-Caribbean people did not regard local community organisations or networks as capable of representing their interests, and would not participate. They considered that the context of institutionalised racism in the health services would impinge upon their participation. This minority group view was unrecognised by those promoting community participation, resulting in inability to include those groups but may bring new ideas and resources. The relationship between community attachment and the ability to mobilise for change needs further research.

Including minority groups

Developing the community field is challenging when groups are not well connected, when there are low levels of community attachment, or when important groups of people are excluded from decision-making processes. This is often the case in communities of place where there are different cultural groups. Even if formal structures are constructed to bring people together, it is difficult to reflect the interests of a diverse and fragmented community (Frankish et al. 2002, p. 1476). Case example 10.7 illustrates this point.

Case example 10.8 is another example of a community where there are divisions between groups and consequent difficulties in getting the community to come together as a whole.

CASE EXAMPLE 10.8

Separate social structures

Source: Taylor 2004, p. 143

In a regional town, the local society clearly separates Aboriginal people from non-Aboriginal. While the populations coexist, there is limited interaction and parallel social structures. The degree of exclusion is high, meaning that most Aboriginal people are neither members of community groups nor asked to attend social events held by non-Aboriginal community members. This social structure limits interaction between the Aboriginal and the non-Aboriginal community, and limits communitywide problem-solving and development. These divisions impact upon the emergence of a community field, as not all the groups can come together.

Including minority groups involves carefully building relationships, understanding how and why groups are currently excluded, and identifying ways that people could be involved. Critical to this process is awareness of how the proposed inclusion strategies may force cultural groups to adapt and deny the significance of their own cultural background (Durie 1994). These are issues that need careful exploration in order to build the community field.

Activity 10.3

Developing the community field

Using Case example 10.8, consider some strategies that community leaders might use to build relationships between Aboriginal and non-Aboriginal people in order to develop the community.

Balancing task and group maintenance functions

Ensuring that the job gets done and at the same time facilitating people working together is an important leadership function. On occasion, these two elements may be in conflict. This is all too common when, for example, a tight deadline for a submission means that one person takes control and gets the submission in on time. Others who offered to be involved are left out, and they may feel that their contributions were not valued.

Small group theory (Johnson and Johnson 2006) uses the concepts of task and group maintenance functions in working together in groups. Task-oriented functions include clarifying the problem, identifying solutions, directing action, and doing things. Group maintenance functions include ensuring inclusion of different ideas, confirming members' contributions, negotiating conflict, and clarifying meaning. In order for a group to work together effectively, both task and group maintenance processes must be attended to.

Usually there are people in a group who have a tendency to focus on task achievement, and there are others who focus on emotional leadership and the process of working together. It is important for leaders to be aware of how both of these aspects are being attended to, and, if necessary, focus on one or other of them.

Practice tip 10.3

It is rare to find leaders who are equally adept at group task and maintenance functions. Be careful of expecting too much of community leaders.

Developing community leadership

Community leadership is complicated and often controversial work. Emotional support for leaders and appropriate opportunities to develop skills are essential. There are a number of programs designed to support an individual's leadership development, as leadership has been a major topic in management (Cacioppe 1998). However, there is less information about *community* leadership training, and therefore exercises presented here have been chosen because they are designed to involve both leaders and their constituents. The exercises focus on the three key areas for leadership presented earlier: finding a common purpose; developing the community field; and balancing task and maintenance functions in group work.

It is important that these exercises here are not seen as a way to address leadership problems, but rather used in an ongoing process that builds on existing skills. For some exercises, it may be useful to have a facilitator who is external to the community and who can take a fresh perspective on the strengths and limitations of current leadership processes.

The exercises can be used with different-sized groups, and can be adjusted to be locally relevant. In most cases, using methods in addition to discussion, such as visual representations and tape recordings, is an option. There is no need for exercises to be followed exactly as they are written here—they are a guide only.

Activity 10.4

Exercises to build a common purpose

A community portrait

Purpose: Developing common themes about the community through pictures.

Participants: Can be used communitywide, or with a particular group in mind. Appropriate when there are diverse CALD groups or those who enjoy working with visual images.

Leadership: Can be facilitated by any leadership group within the community.

Process:

1   Community members are invited to prepare for the workshop by finding pictures that they think represent their community. People may take photos, draw pictures, find newspaper photos, or draw on historical records. Groups may prepare their pictures together.

2   Leaders facilitate people talking about what they represent and collect information.

3   Participants brainstorm themes.

4   A community portrait is designed with pictures grouped around the themes.

Outcomes: Leaders and community members are aware of some common themes about the community that may help in organising community action. The community portrait may be edited and circulated in the community.

Community narratives

Purpose: Sharing stories about the community.

Participants: Can be used communitywide, or with a particular group in mind. It is appropriate when there is a need to bring newer and long-term residents together, and is useful with those groups who like storytelling and reminiscing.

Leadership: Can be facilitated by any leadership group within the community.

Process:

1   Community members are invited to prepare for the workshop by collecting stories about the community. Guidelines about what kinds of stories may be appropriate, such as overcoming adversity or innovation. The stories may be already recorded or they may be written for the occasion.

2   Leaders facilitate people telling their stories.

3   Participants brainstorm what they learnt from the stories and how stories illustrate community strengths or other issues.

Outcomes: Leaders and community members share information about community strengths that may be relevant in organising community action.

Activity 10.5

Building the community field: A community leadership roundtable

Source: adapted from Born 2000: Appendix p. 7

Purpose: The roundtable provides an opportunity to bring diverse community groups together to develop community leadership.

Participants: All community leadership groups are invited to attend, with special attention to those who are not currently active in whole-of-community development.

Leadership: An external facilitator, who is trusted by all groups involved, is preferable. Some community members who attend the roundtable may perceive that they have been excluded from leadership.

Time needed: Two half-days.

Structure: The roundtable is conducted in two phases.

Phase 1: This is a brainingstorming exercise to identify all the community interest groups, networks, and families who may have an interest in community leadership. Strategies to engage with these groups are identified, and planning for the roundtable proceeds with all those who agree to be involved.

Phase 2: The purpose of the day is outlined by the facilitator as a roundtable to assist effective community leadership and development. It is important that the facilitator stresses the positives that are apparent with current community leadership and that the workshop's purpose is to assist this. Questions are discussed in small groups or one large group. In each group, there is a facilitator who asks these questions:

➤ What does community leadership mean to you?
➤ What are the important values in community leadership?
➤ What is your vision for community leadership?
➤ What are the most important things the community can do to work towards effective community leadership?
➤ What will community leadership look like in five years time?

The answers to the future-oriented questions are further discussed in order to develop strategies to address sustainable community leadership.

Outcomes: Links across different community groups, networks, and interest areas are strengthened through discussion of key leadership issues. Practical strategies to address leadership issues are available for implementation.

Activity 10.6

Task and group maintenance functions

Source: adapted from Johnson and Johnson 2006

Purpose: This exercise enables community members to distinguish between task and group maintenance functions in leadership.

Participants: Community members and community leadership groups.

Leadership: Can be facilitated by community members or an external facilitator.

Time needed: Two hours.

Process: Small groups with between six and eight people are organised. Each group has the same task to complete within a specified time. Tasks can be chosen to suit the interest of participants, but should allow for group participation. Examples are:

> drawing a plan for a community park;
> designing a flag or symbol for the community;
> building a structure out of leggo blocks.

One or two observers are chosen in each group. Their role is to observe the problem-solving and group maintenance leadership that is demonstrated in completing the task. Observers give feedback on the leadership process.

Outcome: Participants are aware of task and group maintenance leadership functions as a first step in developing the ability to balance these leadership functions in health and social care development.

SUMMARY

This chapter has put forward a relational view of community leadership as a multi-directional process. According to this perspective, patterns of interaction emerge between community members when some people are exerting influence in order to lead others. This view of leadership is relevant in working with communities where the ability to lead rests on having people join with the leadership. It is dissimilar to organisational leadership where a position in a formal organisation may prescribe leadership.

The key components of community leadership involve identifying a common purpose and then bringing people together across sectors, interest groups, and cultures to work together. It is always difficult to ensure a spread of leaders across the different interest groups in the community, and sometimes too few people wear too many hats. Therefore, capturing people's energy and enthusiasm, and helping ensure that it is appropriately used, is a key leadership challenge. The other important task is to ensure that community leadership is sustainable, and one of the ways to do this is the regular use of activities that bring community people together to reflect on leadership issues.

USEFUL WEBSITES

URP Toolbox: https://www3.secure.griffith.edu.au/03/toolbox/alpha_tool_list.php
Community builders NSW leadership training: http://www.communitybuilders.nsw.gov.au/builder/leaders/aus_lead.html
Department of Local Government and Regional Development Western Australia leadership training: http://www.dlgrd.wa.gov.au/RegionDev/WALeadership.asp
Community Leadership Australia—a not-for-profit organisation: www.communityleadershipaustralia.org
The Oxfam Community Leadership Program: http://www.oxfam.org.au/CLP

CHAPTER 11

Community Planning

Introduction

While there are specific techniques that are useful in community planning, the processes of decision-making, leadership, and forming partnerships discussed in preceding chapters are all crucial elements. The information provided in Chapter 4 about measuring and building community capacity is also important. This chapter explains how these elements come together in community planning, explains the process, and describes some useful techniques, including Rapid Appraisal (Ong et al. 1991), conducting a service audit, and the Delphi survey technique. In addition, two particular types of community planning receive attention—building a community health profile (Rissel and Bracht 1999) and community disaster recovery assessments (Emergency Management Australia 2002).

Community planning for health and social care development

Health and social care development always involves assessment of community needs and capacity at some stage in the process of working with the community. There has been a change of emphasis in health education and human service development from a narrowly conceived needs assessment rooted in 'deficit thinking' to a broader notion of community appraisal. Community planning now involves using multiple methods for collecting information to give a picture not only of community needs, problems, and issues, but also assets and strengths (McKnight and Kretzmann 2005, p. 136).

Collaborative activity is at the heart of community planning, and involves assessing present needs of residents, anticipating future ones, and developing services, programs, facilities, and resources to provide for these (Cheers et al. 2007). Involvement of communities in all aspects of the planning process levers a commitment to the plan, and ensures that the strategies developed will be progressed. The steps may include needs assessment, analysing information, developing strategies, implementation, and evaluating outcomes. These are usually undertaken sequentially. The process may be extensive, collecting information from many sources; or it may be intensive, as in Rapid Appraisal (RA), and used to understand communities' own perceptions of their priority needs (Bar-On and Prinsen 1999).

What do we mean by community planning?

Community planning is an exercise to engage a whole community through its various social fields in identifying achievable goals and strategies for community

TABLE 11.1 Community plan content (adapted from Cheers et al. 2007, p. 52)

Component	Content
Executive summary	Concise summary of the plan, emphasising the vision for the community and key recommendations
Background	Why the plan was formulated; its history; who owns it; how it is legitimated and implemented; how it relates to other local, regional, or State and Federal Government plans
Community health and/ or social care profile	Community history; present social, demographic, health, and infrastructure profile; significant dominant narratives
Vision for the community	Future profile and character of the community
Priority goals, and objectives	Short-term, medium-term, and long-term goals and objectives for the community as a whole and each sector
Strategies for each goal and objective	Preferred strategies; viable alternatives; comparative risk assessments
Performance indicators	Key performance indicators for each goal
Potential resources	Funding—programs; key contacts; strategies Key organisations and people within and outside the community—skills; interests; potential partnerships; suggested lobbying strategies
Related reference material	Local—research, consultancy, and other reports; related plans and historical documents; demographic information, service usage External—e.g., reports; national, state, and regional plans; statistics

health and social care development. A community plan may include a socio-demographic and health profile of the community, a service audit, current health and social care pathways, as well as a vision for the future. It will include priority goals and objectives, strategies to achieve them, performance indicators, timeframes, and potentially useful resources. Table 11.1 (page 217) is an example of the components of a community plan.

Practice tip 11.1   Examples of community plans

Go to the following websites for examples of community plans:

Franklin Harbour District Council:
http://www.franklinharbour.sa.gov.au/webdata/resources/files/
Franklin_Harbour_Strategic_Plan_2006.pdf

City of Port Phillip:
http://www.portphillip.vic.gov.au/new_community_plan.html

For a community plan to have local and external credibility, the power to galvanise action by multiple stakeholders, and be implemented, it must be owned by the community through a local organisation that is recognised as representing the main local interests. It should also be based on sound information, produced with the wide participation of local sectors, groups, and interests, and recognised as speaking for the whole community. When legitimised by the community and relevant government agencies, community plans are powerful instruments that can have a major influence on social, health, and community development.

However, it is important to note that community planning can be a challenging process. The process may bring to light competing local agendas with respect to issues such as service and infrastructure priorities, and these differences have to be negotiated. Plans can also identify gaps in resources, services, and programs that can challenge organisations whose responsibility it is to provide those services. On occasion, the identified gaps that the community sees as important to address may not match the strategic agendas of the relevant government agencies. This makes it difficult to respond to community-identified needs. Therefore it is essential that all the elements of working with communities mentioned previously—partnerships, leadership, and decision-making processes—are in place if the planning process is to be effective and legitimised by key stakeholders.

In spite of the challenges, the benefits of a community-owned local health or social care plan are significant, especially considering the current emphasis on early intervention in health and social problems, and the move to primary health care approaches. A community primary health or social care plan is an important step in stimulating local action.

CASE EXAMPLE 11.1

The neighbourhood community plan

The local neighbourhood centre in association with local government had obtained funding for an inner-city neighbourhood to undertake a community planning initiative. While the neighbourhood had retained its long-term residents, new residential housing developments had brought families and younger people into the area. There were new arrivals from different linguistic and cultural backgrounds, and the local schools were anxious to include these people in their school community. Health professionals were also interested to know more about people's health issues and whether people were aware of the available services.

The neighbourhood centre had employed a community development worker to undertake the planning process, and was keen that community participation be maximised. People thought it was important not only to identify gaps in services and facilities, but also residents' understandings of community strengths. The community plan was to be launched by local government at their annual 'open council' meeting in six months time.

Think about it

➤ If you were the community worker involved in developing the plan, what explanation for conducting the planning exercise would you give to community members?
➤ What components of the planning framework presented above would you include?
➤ Who do you think might be the key community groups, organisations, and individuals who should be involved?
➤ How would the plan be presented at the annual 'open council' meeting?

Practice tip 11.2   Australian Bureau of Statistics Basic Community Profiles

If you are trying to understand the demographics of your community, the ABS Basic Community Profiles are often the best place to start. http://www.abs.gov.au/AUSSTATS/abs@.nsf//web+pages/ Census+Data#BCP

Including community capacity assessments

In developing a community plan, community capacity assessments may be included in two ways. First, the approaches to community capacity assessment described in Chapter 4 may be used. Workshops attended by representatives from different community sectors may be held over several days to audit capacity, using an appropriate quantitative or qualitative framework. If the community plan is looking at development across sectors, then a comprehensive assessment is useful.

If the plan is focusing on a particular aspect, for example developing a health-promotion plan, then another approach is to obtain an assessment of the relevant capacities. For example, in health promotion, the ability to bring sectors together

Activity 11.1

Assessing community capacity to conduct a healthy eating campaign

The promotion of healthy eating as an early intervention strategy to prevent the onset of chronic disease was an important priority for a regional health service. The service was keen to involve other sectors, groups, and community members, but was unsure which resources, networks, and links might be available.

Think about it

➤ How would you assist the regional health service in assessing the capacity the community has to implement a healthy eating campaign?

Practice tip 11.3   Resources to assess capacity

The resources provided by the NSW government community builders' site are useful to assess capacity. http://www.communitybuilders. nsw.gov.au/getting_started/needs

is important, as is the ability to mobilise the community field, and to identify the resources and networks that are available to work on the tasks both from within and external to the community. The nine capacity domains for health promotion, discussed in Chapter 4—participation, leadership, organisational structures, problem assessment, resource mobilisation, 'asking why?', links with others, role of outside agents, and program management—are important to assess (Labonte and Laverack 2001, p. 116). This can be done using community workshops, focused group discussions, and individual interviews. Some of the techniques described later in the chapter will be useful in this process.

A community health profile

This is a form of community planning that provides a snapshot of a community's health. Although the purpose of community health profiles varies considerably, the following information is usually included (Nelson 2001):

➤ demographic information about the community;
➤ health status information that is routinely collected locally, regionally, and nationally;
➤ information about health service usage and access;
➤ qualitative information about attitudes to health and factors that affect participation in health activities; and
➤ community strengths.

The community profile is best done as a partnership between communities and health planners, in order to use existing information and to determine what new information needs to be collected. Existing information may be supplemented by one-off data collection. Community health planning is most useful if there is some comparative information—either with other populations nationally or regionally, or with the same community over time (Wright and Walley 1998).

Health status information

The bulk of information used in a community health profile comes from information that is routinely collected, either from national, regional, or local sources. Often in small communities of place or of interest, specific information about the community is difficult to obtain. Health planners can assist in overcoming this problem. Routine information may be obtained from:

➤ local hospital inpatient and outpatient records;

➤ health profiles produced by regional health services;

➤ state-based health information, such as pregnancy outcomes data and immunisation status; and

➤ national health reports, for example *The Health and Welfare of Australia's Aboriginal and Torres Strait Islander Peoples* (Trewin and Madden 2003).

The types of information that may be available in a health profile include a health and wellness outcomes profile (morbidity and mortality data); a health risk profile (including behavioural, social and environmental risks); and a survey of current health-promotion policies, programs, and activity (Rissel and Bracht 1999).

If there are difficulties in obtaining relevant health information about a specific community, it may be necessary to supplement the information through one-off surveys, focus groups, or interviews with health professionals. Whatever method is chosen, it is important to make the data collection process as simple and rigorous as possible to ensure that the process can be replicated to show changes over time.

Health service usage and access

Usually it is possible to obtain some health service usage information at the community level, but again, it will be important to seek advice on how to go about this. Health planners are the first port of call. Monash University Rural Health School provides health service profiles for rural Victorian regions (see http://www.med.monash.edu.au/srh/resources). For information about general practice activity in Australia, see *General Practice in Australia 2004* (Commonwealth of Australia 2005), available on line at http://www.health.gov.au/internet/wcms/Publishing.nsf/Content/pcd-publications-gpinoz2004

One way to understand about health services access from a consumer or community perspective is to undertake a pathways mapping exercise. This involves a group of community members brainstorming the steps involved in accessing health care for a particular condition. These are recorded and displayed as a map. Usually the map includes the health care or other agencies that people could speak to about the problem, who they might be referred to, the steps in the

Practice tip 11.4   Sources of health service usage information

Here are some potential health service usage data that may be relevant and possible to obtain from your state health department:

➤ occupancy rates and discharges from local hospitals;
➤ utilisation of specialists who are available in the local community;
➤ patterns of attendance at outpatient facilities;
➤ attendance at community health centres; and
➤ information from general practice services indicating attendance rates.

referral process, and where the services are located. Pathway mapping is most useful to reveal the complexity of the health care system when there are multiple referral points and different service options.

Attitudes to health and participation in health activities

It is important to start with information that is already available on the topic. Generally, communities have conducted some kind of assessment of health

Activity 11.2

Community planning for health service delivery

A regional community is interested in having a community mental health plan. Your role is to organise a brainstorming group to map pathways into health care for people with depression. This is important to determine the adequacy and relevance of current services.

Think about it

➤ Whom would you invite to be part of the group?
➤ What resources would you need?

issues that can provide the foundation for further information gathering. If additional information is to be obtained, it is important to ask questions that provoke meaningful discussion and be helpful to communities in understanding their health. Focus groups and key informant interviews, along with surveys, are methods commonly used to gain this information, and there are several standardised instruments. Ask your local health planner for advice.

Planning for community recovery following a disaster

Effective recovery from a disaster, either a natural disaster, such as a bushfire, or a catastrophic event, such as a plane crash or terrorist attack, involves enabling and supportive processes to assist individuals, families, and communities to attain a proper level of functioning. The objective of disaster recovery planning is to provide effective and efficient coordination and delivery of programs, in collaboration with communities, to assist and hasten recovery. The disaster-recovery plan is a key element detailing how information, specialist services, and resources will be provided.

Most communities will have a disaster-recovery plan as a component of an emergency management plan prepared collaboratively by local, regional, or state emergency management authorities. They may have a local community recovery committee, and conduct regular training programs and exercises. However, the aftermath of a disaster places enormous strains on community functioning and, in particular, on community leadership processes and decision-making. This is why preparedness is essential.

The components of recovery management planning are comprehensively dealt with in the Australian Emergency Services Manual 10 (Emergency Management Australia 2002). This section provides a brief overview of the key components of the recovery plan and some of the aspects of community functioning that will be affected following a disaster.

The community recovery plan

The recovery plan is prepared in association with emergency management authorities, with contributions from key government agencies, including police, local government, health services, and non-government community agencies. The roles and functions of each of the contributing agencies and the disaster recovery manager are clearly identified in the plan. The purpose of this is to

CASE EXAMPLE 11.2

The disaster recovery committee

In a regional centre, the disaster recovery committee met monthly. Membership included the state government department with the responsibility for recovery functions, the police, Lifeline, the emergency housing agency and the Red Cross. Meetings involved updating members on disaster recovery training options, reviewing the recovery plan, and checking contact details. The committee had provided recovery functions following tropical cyclones and was well aware of the importance of maintaining preparedness.

The regional centre had a recovery plan that included roles and responsibilities with regard to the following functions:

➤ needs assessment;
➤ providing information including establishing a one-stop shop;
➤ emergency housing arrangements;
➤ provision of food and clothing;
➤ one-on-one counselling;
➤ debriefing;
➤ provision of financial assistance and advice on insurance; and
➤ longer term recovery.

ensure that every agency and organisation knows its role following a disaster, what resources will be required to fulfil the role, and that these resources are in place. It is essential that the plan be kept up to date and that this occurs through coordinated emergency management.

Needs assessment

The type of assessment that will be conducted depends on the nature of the event, its size, and its effects. Needs will be assessed as soon as possible after the emergency, but the assessment may be supplemented once the full impact of the event is known. The assessment looks at the effects of the event on the community, considering its demography and the resources it has to deal with the event. Because the context is continually changing, a needs assessment is conducted in association with local people.

Providing information

Often a one-stop shop providing all types of information and assistance will be established in a predetermined location. This aids service coordination and avoids people having to travel to various locations and telling their story several times. It also creates access to services, such as counselling and health services, which may not have been thought of as able to provide assistance.

The processes through which information will be provided to community members will be planned. Public meetings, television community service announcements, emergency phone-ins, press releases, and radio are all avenues for information dissemination. The arrangements for using these mediums and the contact numbers will be in the plan.

Emergency service provision

It is important that the community disaster-recovery plan identifies the agencies that will provide emergency services. Usually federal, state, and local government all have responsibilities, and it is how these services will be coordinated, what will be provided, and who will be involved that will be outlined in the plan.

Activity 11.3

Community recovery planning following a cyclone

A small community of approximately 300 people had been severely affected by a tropical cyclone. Several public buildings including the bank had lost part of their roofs, and about one-third of the town's houses were damaged by wind and the flood waters that followed the cyclone. The river on which the town was located had flooded, making access to the centre of the town from surrounding areas difficult. Staff from the agency responsible for disaster recovery had to be airlifted into the community to carry out a needs assessment, set up a one-stop shop, and help with emergency service provision.

Think about it

➤ In establishing the information one-stop shop, what needs to be considered about its location?
➤ How will community members find out about it?
➤ What services could be provided at the location?

Local agencies will also be responsible for some aspects, such as counselling and emergency provision of food and clothing. Volunteers associated with community agencies may have important roles in emergency service provision.

Community recovery planning concepts

Experience gained from a variety of different kinds of events suggests that recovery is optimised when individuals and communities affected actively participate in its management (Emergency Management Australia 2002, p. 107). However, the impact of a large-scale natural disaster such as an earthquake, flood, or bushfire on community functioning is enormous, creating a state of crisis and cleavages between social networks both internally and with outside groups and individuals. It is important to understand how emergencies disrupt the patterns of social interaction and communication.

De-bonding

The interactional understanding of communities presented in Chapter 2 stresses the importance of social interactions, social organisation, and horizontal and vertical ties in community functioning. In a disaster, the usual patterns of social bonds and interactions are suspended in favour of new interactions and relationships. This phenomenon is known as 'de-bonding' and involves suspending or setting aside the bonds that constitute the fabric of social life. It is a central concept in community recovery planning, as de-bonding, even for a short time, has repercussions on the community (Emergency Management Australia 2002, p. 115).

The effect of the disaster is to separate people physically and emotionally. For example, people are relocated to emergency shelters if fire or floods threaten their homes. This separates people from their usual social supports, including friends or family. Communication to the affected areas is usually disrupted, with the result that people most affected by the disaster are separated from the rest of the community. Consequently, the usual systems of social organisation and community functioning are affected, and this is highly threatening. Newly established task-focused networks, essential to assist recovery, replace the usual interaction patterns.

Fusion

The social processes where communities organise around the aftermath of a disaster is known as 'fusion' (Emergency Management Australia 2002 p. 118). Intense social connectedness is activated as people re-establish communication, support each other, and share experiences. Depending on the extent and type of the disaster, the community may be united through participation in immediate concrete tasks and create new 'fused' community processes that are different from the pre-disaster networks.

There may be heightened community solidarity at this time, with increased intolerance of outsiders who did not experience the disaster, and there may be a reduction in the social separation between community groups that were previously marginalised. There is a sense of the community working together that is reinforced by media coverage and the profile that is achieved immediately following the disaster.

Re-bonding

Community cohesion achieved through the disaster is not long-lasting. Over time, the disaster recovery tasks become less intense as the need to perform everyday tasks returns. Schools and shops reopen and public transport is reinstated. Therefore, people must withdraw from the recovery-oriented networks to their usual social networks. The process of withdrawing may produce tension and conflict as the community 'winds down' from the disaster effort. There may be questions about the accuracy of information provided during the disaster and distribution of resources. Leaders may be blamed for inadequacies in services and resources, and these factors may contribute to the weakening of pre-disaster community networks and social organisation. Groups may feel they have been isolated and receive less service, resulting in social conflict (Carroll et al. 2006, p. 269).

CASE EXAMPLE 11.3

Bushfires on the Lower Eyre Peninsula 2005

Source: Burning Issues Exhibition Handbook, 2005. The exhibition was curated by Jo McLeay and supported by ETSA and Country Arts SA **http://www.etsautilities.com.au/default.jsp?xcid=946**

Jillian Parker, the Chairperson of Burning Issues Exhibition Committee, describes the bushfires:

> On January 11th 2005, the most destructive fire ever seen in this area devastated Southern Eyre Peninsula. The power, the intensity, the noise, the speed, and the devastation left behind, was very hard to comprehend and those who were involved may never fully recover from its wrath.

Nine lives were lost, including four children. People lost their homes, their stock, equipment, property fences, gardens, and their livelihood. The environment was ravaged. There was an extensive disaster recovery effort. Volunteers from all over South Australia travelled to the area to help people rebuild their properties and pick up their lives. A one-stop shop provided information, resources, and counselling. Effective networking occurred between those affected, agencies, volunteers, and communities. Immediately following the disaster, these networks replaced the usual patterns of interaction, which had been disrupted by the fire.

After some months families decided whether they would rebuild or leave the community, the one-stop shop closed, and communities tried to get back to normal. But normality was difficult to achieve for some communities. There was ongoing distress about the loss of life and debate about the response to the fire and its causation.

One way communities became proactive in handling their grief and demonstrating their strength was by producing an exhibition using the media of visual art, photography, and written and spoken accounts. The catalogue 'Burning Issues', produced for the exhibition commemorating the bushfires, is dedicated to the nine who lost their lives and to the suffering families, friends, and the ravaged environment.

Think about it

➤ What were some of the effects of the bushfire on community networks?
➤ What new networks might have formed to acknowledge the personal tragedy, the destruction of property, and the devastation of the environment?

Techniques for community planning

In this section, we discuss techniques for gathering information to contribute to community plans and community health profiles. Not all of these techniques will be used in any one planning process, but all of them have value.

Rapid Appraisal

There are a number of terms that are used similarly to describe this approach, including 'Participatory Rural Appraisal' (PRA) (Gona et al. 2006), and 'Rapid Rural Appraisal' (RRA) (Melville 1993). In this section, we use the term 'Rapid

Appraisal' (RA) to describe a variety of methods and techniques practised in rural and urban locations, and having the following characteristics in common:

➤ greater speed compared with conventional methods of analysis;
➤ working 'in the field';
➤ an emphasis on learning directly from the local inhabitants;
➤ a semi-structured, multidisciplinary approach with room for flexibility and innovation;
➤ an emphasis on producing timely insights, hypotheses or 'best bets' rather than final truths or fixed recommendations. (Ong et al. 1991, p. 910)

RA is a comprehensive approach to community planning developed in relatively socio-economically deprived communities. It enables identification of health and social care issues with cooperation between communities, practitioners, and local government within a short timeframe. It heightens community engagement and enables locally driven service development. According to Bar-On and Prinsen (1999, p. 277), RA is a '[f]amily of methods that enables communities to assemble with formal service providers, identify and analyse critical elements of their life in their own idioms, and plan and carry through feasible changes'.

The six principles that guide RA have been adapted from those presented by Bar-On and Prinsen (1999). First, all activities are undertaken as an opportunity to learn about community issues, and there is active stakeholder participation. Second, facilitators and community leaders draw information from the widest possible range of groups and external agencies that have knowledge about the community, using a range of methods, tools, and activities. Third, goals and methodologies are flexible, as they are revised in response to an increasing understanding of community needs. Fourth, RA identifies and builds on strengths and assets rather than starting with weaknesses and deficits. Fifth, data-gathering is based around listening to people, recognising that people know their own needs. Finally, in the interests of having information back for the community quickly, facilitators use a commonsense approach in analysing the data, and look for corroboration and discrepancies between different information sets.

The six steps in RA are adapted from those Bar-On and Prinsen (1999) suggest. They can be modified as necessary. It is important to have facilitators from community leadership groups and interested key stakeholders to guide the process.

1 *Preparation* (3–5 days): Facilitators provide information to potential participants and sensitise them to the reasons for, and the outcomes desired from, the planning process.
2 *Data-gathering* (4–6 days): A range of methods are used to collect information, including workshops, interviews, non-participant observation, and collection

CASE EXAMPLE 11.4

Rapid Appraisal for the community health plan

Source: adapted from Taylor et al. in press

As part of a new funding initiative, an Aboriginal community had to undertake a planning process to determine how they wanted to improve maternal and antenatal care. There was a tight timeframe of one month in which to conduct the planning exercise. The community had an Aboriginal health service with strong connections with 'mainstream' health care providers.

The community decided that it would use an RA process to gather information, determine priorities, and devise the strategies and indicators. It chose this method because of the short timeframe and because it had key stakeholders in the health service to assist with obtaining relevant information. It also had a mothers, and babies, group that met regularly and was eager to get involved. There was a keen interest in improving maternal and child health as fundamental to community wellbeing.

Think about it

➤ If you were one of the facilitators chosen to help the process with the Aboriginal community, what steps would you suggest in conducting the RA?

➤ Who do you think might be the key community groups, organisations and individuals who should be involved?

➤ What kinds of information should be collected?

➤ How would the information be presented to the community?

of written records (Brown et al. 2006). Participants 'picture' their community and how they want it to develop.

3   *Synthesis* (1–2 days): Facilitators and elected community representatives group the information into broad issue categories, such as education, health, and transport, and present it to the community for discussion, modification, and verification.

4   *Ranking* (1–2 days): Workshop participants prioritise issues with key stakeholders involved. Commitment to change increases when participants and key stakeholders negotiate together.

5   *Preparing and adopting a community action plan* (3–4 days): Participants prepare the plan as they devise strategies to tackle the identified issues. It is then presented to the general community and service providers.

6   *Implementation and monitoring*: Carried out by government agencies, various joint governmental and non-governmental committees, and local community workers.

Surveys

Surveys are a common research tool to collect information on people's views about community health and social care issues, needs and priorities, satisfaction with current arrangements, and patterns of service usage. Depending on the purpose of the survey, the target may be the entire community or a particular group.

Once the purpose of the survey is clear, then a decision can be made as to how information will be collected, whether it will be self-administered or delivered via face-to-face or telephone interviews, posted out, or emailed. Questions will be carefully constructed so that the meaning is clear, there are no 'double-barrelled'

CASE EXAMPLE 11.5

Interest in the Internet

The community centre in a regional neighbourhood had heard from some older people that they were interested in accessing the Internet and learning more about how they could use it. There was an opportunity to obtain a grant to set up access to the Internet and provide training for older people in its use. The community centre wanted to know more about people's levels of interest, whether they already had access to the Internet and whether or not training would be useful.

Think about it

➤ What would be the reasons that a survey might be appropriate to obtain the information?

➤ What would be the reasons that a survey might not be useful?

➤ If a survey was conducted, what type should be used; email, postal, face-to-face interview, or an opportunistic survey at a place where older people might gather?

➤ How would you feed back your information?

Practice tip 11.5 Information about surveys

Useful information about using a survey for planning is available at the URP Toolbox: https://www3.secure.griffith.edu.au/03/toolbox/display_tool.php?pk1=16

questions, and the information obtained can be easily collated. Surveys are always piloted, that is, tested with individuals who share characteristics of the target group. This is a way to ensure that the questions are unambiguous, that there are not too many questions, and the method for recording responses is appropriate.

Opportunistic surveys are those that ask people to answer questions or complete answers on a survey sheet when they are at public places, such as shopping centres or sporting events. While opportunistic surveys are of value when timelines for obtaining information are tight, usually they involve a convenience sample. This means that information is only obtained from those people available on the day, and it is difficult to draw conclusions about the views of the community as a whole.

Activity 11.4

The hotline regarding alcohol use

Several regional communities were interested in knowing more about patterns of alcohol use, especially among younger adults. High schools in the region suspected that alcohol use was widespread among students, but their information was anecdotal. A telephone hotline was suggested where people would be encouraged to talk about patterns of alcohol use and whether or not they thought it was impacting on their own or others' wellbeing.

Think about it

➤ What would be the purpose in conducting a telephone hotline in this situation?
➤ If a hotline was to be conducted, who would answer the phones?
➤ How could the hotline be publicised?
➤ How would the information obtained be fed back to the community?
➤ What use could be made of the information?

Telephone hotlines

This technique is appropriate when information is required about a sensitive topic, such as sexual abuse or domestic violence, and it is thought that having an opportunity to talk anonymously over the phone may encourage contributions (Queensland Domestic Violence Task Force 1988). Its success relies on effective promotion, usually through media releases, in the target community. It must have a telephone number that can be accessed for the cost of a local call, and it is essential that anonymity be maintained. For this reason, and because of the cost and level of organisation involved, it is most commonly used to gain information at the state or national level.

The hotline uses trained people who are conversant with the topic area, and non-identifying information is collected on a survey form. It is important to have a back-up telephone counselling facility, such as Lifeline, available to refer people to if there are ongoing issues arising from the telephone call.

Delphi technique

The Delphi research technique is useful to help bring opinions and views together through several rounds of discussion and reflection, resulting in a consensus view. It is useful in the following situations:

➤ when there are diverse perspectives on the topic area or there is little known;
➤ when there is value in conducting several rounds of information-sharing between experts in order to fully explore the topic and reach consensus;
➤ when face-to-face workshops or discussions are difficult, given the experts' location or time commitments;
➤ when there are experts and they are available and willing to be involved.

The Delphi technique requires a highly skilled facilitator who is trained in research techniques, such as clarifying a research question, managing information, and understanding and being able to detect consensus in participants' views. It uses people who are 'expert' in the topic area. The term 'expert' does not necessarily mean possessing professional expertise. For example, if the Delphi method were being used to explore strategies for improved entry to tertiary education, then young adults who had experienced the education system may be involved, as well as secondary and tertiary education sector representatives. From a community perspective, using a Delphi technique can be particularly appropriate when experts can be engaged through email exchanges. This enables international and national expertise to be obtained.

The steps below may all be relevant in using the Delphi technique, but they need not necessarily be conducted in this order. The technique is iterative, with each round of discussion informing the next until the issue is clarified. The steps are adapted from Hasson et al. (2000, p. 1013).

1   Clarify the problem or issue to be discussed and how consensus will be reached.
2   Decide who would be appropriate to involve as experts and their preferred method of involvement—electronic, email, or written information delivered by fax.
3   Inform participants of what they will be asked to do, how much time it will take, and what use will be made of the information they provide.
4   Decide what type of information will be obtained—qualitative, quantitative or both.
5   Decide how the information will be analysed.

CASE EXAMPLE 11.6

Increasing evidence-based practice

There is an international movement to encourage health and social care professionals to use the best available evidence from research in day-to-day practice. While professionals have embraced the concept, there are difficulties of accessing the best available evidence and using it. Although there is a wealth of information about implementing evidence-based practice, expert opinion is divided as to which are the most appropriate strategies to increase its uptake.

A large health service was keen to engage staff, consumers, and private practitioners in increasing evidence-based practice. It decided to use a Delphi survey technique to determine the most effective strategies for encouraging uptake among the different practitioner groups. It also wanted to investigate whether or not consumers should receive information about evidence-based practice so that they might support the moves to this type of practice.

Think about it

➤   What do you think is the problem or issue to be discussed?
➤   Who do you think might be the 'experts' in discussing this problem or issue?
➤   What resources do you think might be needed to conduct the exercise?
➤   How would you define 'consensus', considering the aim of the exercise?
➤   How would you present the final results?

6   Decide what questions will be asked in the first round. Usually these are open-ended to ensure the full range of opinions to emerge, but questions must be carefully phrased to enable you to compare information.

Perhaps the most important phase in using the Delphi technique is the data collection and analysis. This involves the discovery of opinions, the process of determining the most important issues, and collating views into themes.

In the first round of analysis, information about each issue is grouped together using a software package such as QSR N6 or similar. These groupings (preserving participants' wording) are organised, and become the information for the second round. At this stage, the information may be complemented by relevant literature.

Subsequent rounds of discussion are analysed to identify emerging consensus and divergence, noting the change in participants' opinions. The skills of the facilitator are critical to this process. If communities require help in conducting a Delphi technique, it may be appropriate to form a partnership with a University, where research or teaching staff may have expertise in this technique.

Focused group discussion

Focus groups are guided group discussions to gather opinions and ideas about a topic (Patton 1990). They use a topic guide, which is list of relevant issues that will be discussed. Focused group discussions are useful in all types of community planning where it is important to canvass a range of views and engage with community members. However, they can be used inappropriately if they are seen as a quick and inexpensive way to gather information, as they require expert facilitation and appropriate analysis of the information obtained.

The point of choosing a focus group over individual interviews or a survey is that group processes 'spark' new ideas about a topic being presented, and good facilitation enables deeper exploration of relevant points. They are most useful when it is possible to select people who can provide a range of views about a topic. They are less useful in gaining information about controversial topics that people may be unwilling to talk about in a group situation. This is especially the case in small communities of place or of interest, when participants may know each other, and a lack of anonymity may result in vigilance in discussion. The other problem with focus groups is that the phenomenon of group contagion may occur— people who become dominant in the discussion may spread their ideas forcefully across the group, and others may be less likely to present contrasting views.

Focused group discussion requires a topic guide, and this is developed considering the issues that it is important to gather information about. Then, given the topics, the participants are chosen along with a suitable venue and a facilitator. A method of recording the discussion is essential, and how this is to occur must be decided in association with the participants. It is usual to send back summaries of the discussion to those who participated.

Activity 11.5

Collecting views about the local park

A focus group is to be held to obtain views about the amenities required in a local park. What would be the topics for the focus group? Who should be invited?

Public meeting[1]

A public meeting is one strategy to create a broader public awareness of an issue. It is an open forum that all members of a community have an opportunity to attend and voice their opinions. Considerations such as the timing of the meeting, where it is held, making access easy, and good facilitation, are important to ensure that it is accessible.

A public meeting can be run for a variety of purposes, including raising awareness about an issue, obtaining information from participants about a topic, to give information, or to plan a strategy. It is particularly useful in health and social care development in making what is usually a private issue public. For example, an Aboriginal community in a rural town held an open meeting to publicise the strategies they were implementing to address family violence, which was previously treated as a private issue. They made sure that all relevant community groups were aware that the meeting was on and that they were invited (Taylor, Cheers, Weetra et al. 2004). As a result of the meeting, the issue was opened up for public debate.

A public meeting can involve a whole community and therefore have a large number of attendees, or it can be focused on a particular target group and be quite small. Whatever its size or topic, it is well publicised through local press releases and is held at a time thought to be convenient for those who wish to attend. Facilities for people who are visually or hearing-impaired need to be considered, and child care and transport may need to be available.

Usually a public meeting is facilitated by someone who is conversant with the topic and who is respected by those who will attend. Unless the meeting is well facilitated, those perceived as having power within the community or those who are most articulate may dominate the meeting. The agenda of the meeting should be clear and made available beforehand.

The meeting venue is important. In some situations, holding a meeting outdoors with a meal provided might be appropriate. For more formal meetings, a venue that is well known, easy to access, comfortable, and the right size for the number of attendees may be preferred. If visual aids such as a PowerPoint presentation or overheads are to be used, then an outside venue may not work well.

CASE EXAMPLE 11.7

Getting support for the volunteer program

A regional community had relatively large numbers of young families because of the defence base that was located there. Many of these families were 'on transfer' and consequently were distanced from their usual support networks. A church organisation had obtained 'one-off' funding to implement a volunteer program where older adults act as 'grandparents', or supports, to the families who were new to town. The program was highly regarded and well used. However, funding was coming to an end and the church organisation had thought of holding a public meeting to lobby for community support to seek renewal of funding.

Think about it

➤ What would the purpose of a public meeting be?
➤ Who should be targeted to attend a public meeting?
➤ Who should facilitate the meeting?
➤ Where should it be held?

Service audit

The purpose of a service audit is to find out what services and care processes are currently available and to rate their adequacy and relevance to people in the community. Information gathered is used to assess service strengths and gaps. A service audit is usually conducted in sectors, for example health services or services for those with a disability. How the sector is defined is important. Auditing health services using a holistic perspective on health will involve noting services related to socio-emotional wellbeing provided from outside the health sector. By contrast, a service audit of acute health services will involve primarily the health sector.

A service audit is usually conducted using a template in order to obtain standardised information. It may be administered as a postal survey, collected through face-to-face interviews, or at a regular meeting of the sector that is being audited. Information may be collected about service availability, whether or not services are meeting demand, and the perceived level of service adequacy. It is always important to make clear the purpose of the audit, ensure that the questions are directly related to the purpose, and that respondents know what is to happen with the information that is collected.

Practice tip 11.6

Service audit checklist

➤ Service name
➤ Key functions
➤ Target group
➤ Level of intervention, primary, secondary or tertiary
➤ Hours of operation
➤ Location
➤ Access (disability access, parking, public transport availability, child care)
➤ Staffing levels and staff roles
➤ Community involvement
➤ Complaints mechanism
➤ Types of data collection
➤ Evaluation method

Activity 11.6

Auditing financial support services

Reflecting on the components of a service audit above, what components do you think could be included in an audit of the health and human services sector to determine what services are available to those who are experiencing financial hardship?

Note

1   This information is adapted from the Community Toolbox.

SUMMARY

This chapter presents community planning as a process involving multiple methods for collecting information to give a picture not only of community needs, problems, and issues, but also assets and strengths. All of the skills described in the previous chapter, such as decision-making, developing partnerships, and leadership, are essential in community planning. The planning process may be extensive or it may be a snapshot of an aspect of a community's functioning or service arrangements at a particular time.

A community plan may include a socio-demographic and health profile of the community, a service audit, current health and social care pathways, as well as a vision for the entire community. It will include priority goals and objectives, strategies to achieve them, performance indicators, timeframes, and potentially useful resources.

A community health profile provides a snapshot of a community's health. The following information can be included in a community health profile:

➤ demographic information about the community;
➤ health status information that is routinely collected locally, regionally, and nationally;
➤ information about health service usage;
➤ qualitative information about attitudes to health and factors that affect participation in health activities; and
➤ community strengths.

Another type of community plan is the community disaster recovery plan. This plan is prepared in association with the key government agencies, including police, local government, health services, and NGOs. It is essential that the community recovery plan is kept up to date, and this occurs through a coordinated emergency management approach.

There are a number of techniques that can be used in undertaking community planning exercises, and Rapid Appraisal is useful when there is a need for community involvement and a planning outcome within a short timeframe. Other information-collecting methods, such as surveys, Delphi technique, telephone hotlines, focused group discussions, public meetings, and conducting a service audit, can all be used.

USEFUL WEBSITES

Planning resources

Emergency Management Australia provides useful information on a wide range of
topics including a set of manuals: http://ema.gov.au

The URP Toolbox has information about surveys and focus groups: https://www3.
secure.griffith.edu.au/03/toolbox

Community plans

The Franklin Harbour District Council local government strategic plan based on
a community planning process: http://www.franklinharbour.sa.gov.au/
webdata/resources/files/Franklin_Harbour_Strategic_Plan_2006.pdf

City of Port Phillip community planning process: http://www.portphillip.vic.gov.
au/new_community_plan.html

Health plans

South Australian Aboriginal Health Partnership Substance Misuse Plan: http://
www.ahcsa.org.au/media/docs/substance_misuse.pdf

Spencer Gulf Rural Health School Primary Health Care Research Capacity Building
plan: http://www.phcred-sa.org.au/pdf/SGRHS%20Business%20Plan07.pdf

Information sources

Monash University Rural Health School resources for health planning in Victorian
communities: http://www.med.monash.edu.au/srh/resources/

Australian Bureau of Statistics Basic community profiles: http://www.abs.gov.au/
AUSSTATS/abs@.nsf//web+pages/Census+Data#BCP

Cochrane Collaboration Informed Health: http://www.informedhealthonline.com/
index.en.html

CHAPTER 12

Building Knowledge

Introduction

This final chapter presents information about building the evidence-base about working with communities in community health and social care development. All aspects of working with communities that have been discussed in the previous chapters—planning, building partnerships and decision-making—require information to guide practice. In turn, practice is a good source of information if it is carefully collected. This chapter argues that we need to research aspects of community health and social care development in collaboration with communities in order to build knowledge. The chapter covers the following topics:

➤ building an evidence base in community health and social care development;
➤ how communities can participate in research activities;[1]
➤ participatory Action Research (PAR); and
➤ how to do program evaluation with communities.

Building an evidence-base

The Aspen Institute (Auspos and Kubisch 2004, p. 6) has argued that 'across the field we need to dig deeper around some key questions [about community development], draw on some different sources of evidence and develop a broader knowledge base that goes beyond formal evaluations of programs and initiatives'. This means not only evaluating the program, intervention, or service, but also examining the contextual factors that affect them, and aspects of the process of working with the community to get the program started and to keep it running.

The end result of collecting this information systematically is a body of knowledge available for general use about aspects of community health and social care development. Why programs work well in some communities and not in others, what level of involvement can communities have in different types of decision-making, and the community-level factors that affect program sustainability are all questions that need to be answered. Building knowledge means that there is more information available for practitioners.

Increasing the evidence-base for practice

There is a worldwide movement supporting the implementation of evidence-based practice in all caring disciplines, including nursing, social work, and medicine. In the latter discipline, Sackett (1997, p. 3) provides a definition of evidence-based medicine as being 'the conscientious, explicit, and judicious use of the best available evidence in making decisions about the care of individual patients'. Evidence-based practice in health and social care policy is similar, involving selecting and appraising research to use to inform policy.

While practitioners may be supportive of a move to use evidence, there are constraints to this in practice (McCarthy and Hegney 1998). One of the most serious problems is the gaps in evidence about the complex processes in community health and social care development, such as achieving inclusive decision-making, developing effective partnerships, and sustaining community leadership.

In order to improve practice, and the policy that supports practice, there is national and international attention to building the evidence base about social care and community health. An excellent example of a practical program to help this is the Primary Health Care Research, Evaluation and Development (PHCRED) (http://www.phcris.org.au/phcred/index.php). This program aims to expand the pool of primary health care researchers, to generate more evidence of relevance to primary health care, and to support well-informed primary health care policy and practice.

CASE EXAMPLE 12.1

Research into suicide prevention

A general practitioner (GP) had been worried for some time about the number of suicides that had been occurring in the area. Community members had discussed the issue, and everybody agreed it was imperative to try to address the problem. The GP had contacts with a university that had a Research Capacity Building Initiative (RCBI) and approached the staff to support research. The community decided that it would like the University to help with the research design and the analysis of the information. Through working together, community members found out that there were several aspects of their preventative work that could be 'fine-tuned' to improve what they were doing to address the problem. The GP and community members presented the results at a national conference, and made links with other communities that were facing similar problems.

Strategies to achieve these aims include assisting practitioners, consumers, and communities build research skills in order that they may explore issues of relevance in a systematic way. Increasing awareness of research and its value at the community level is a related strategy, as is the development of a research workforce in order to address the gaps in evidence.

Most departments of general practice in Australia, as well as university departments of rural health, are funded under the PHCRED Strategy's Research Capacity Building Initiative (RCBI), under which research training and support is delivered, especially to local practitioners and communities. Staff who work under this program are available to provide advice on building research capacity, may provide access to formal research training programs, and may be available to give advice about specific research projects. For more information about the PHCRED program, please access the website for contact details in your area.

Practice tip 12.1

For an example of a PHCRED program go to http://www.phcred-sa.org.au

Community participation in research

In Case example 12.1, community people were involved in researching a serious problem. Interviews were conducted with knowledgeable people about the social and economic issues that they thought might be important. They also obtained demographic and health and social care service usage information. In addition, the university provided reports and journal articles about suicide in communities to provide a clearer picture of the problem nationally and the approaches that were being used. Throughout the process, the university, the GP, counsellors, hospital staff, and members of community organisations worked together to unravel the research process so that people would not be scared off by what could be seen as a rather intimidating technical process (Taylor and Fuller 2004).

People do research in their everyday lives when they want to find a solution to a problem, and while this was a complex topic, the process was the same—systematically collecting information and making sense of it. Through working together, the people demystified the research process, and everyone could participate (Wadsworth 1997). Research and program development are intertwined, with each informing the other (Ife and Tesoriero 2006, p. 309).

Another area where community members can be involved is in evaluating programs and services. Increasingly, evaluation is seen as a collaborative activity between communities and evaluators. Community members who have firsthand experience of a program may be best placed to produce information about the program's functioning and usefulness. In any case, it is imperative that there be constant feedback from communities about program strengths and limitations. Usually there are formal mechanisms for obtaining this type of feedback, but community participation in evaluation of community programs should be seen as mandatory (Cohen and Uphoff 1977).

Activity 12.1

Community involvement in evaluation

Think of a program or service with which you are familiar. What are the ways that community members could get involved in evaluating the program or service?

Does research require specialist skills?

Research can become an ordinary activity done by ordinary people—not only something that universities, specialists, or experts do. Community health and social care development is not so complex or vague that it is impossible to research, and if people are interested, there are research training courses available. However, there are two important provisos when we promote the idea of research as an ordinary activity. First, we need to be very clear about what it is we are trying to find out, and second, it is imperative to work with a team and obtain advice from people who are skilled in research.

Practice tip 12.2

Community-based research resources: University of Washington
http://sphcm.washington.edu/research/community.asp

One research framework that enables a team approach using a mix of contributions and expertise is called Participatory Action Research (PAR) (Stringer 1999). This is a research framework that involves collaborative planning, taking action, and reflecting on the action in an ongoing cycle. It is useful in understanding both the context, processes involved, and outcomes of community health and social care development.

Participatory action research

Participatory action research (PAR) is a way of involving participants in addressing a real-life problem through a research process. It is a research and evaluation framework rather than a methodology in its own right, and can be used with all types of research including both quantitative (involving measurement through obtaining numerical values that can be analysed statistically) and qualitative (an interpretative approach to understand social phenomena). The challenge is to maintain rigour in the research process while providing solutions to address a real-life problem.

The framework involves a cycle of joint planning, action, and reflection in continuous loops, with each of the steps in the loops informing the next, and so in. In PAR, unlike other research approaches, there is no push to get the research process right at the outset. For example, sometimes research is about complex problems, and we don't really know exactly how to start. We can test out our ideas about which questions to ask, and then we can adjust these as we learn more. The principle of PAR is that we go through a number of planning, action, and reflection cycles. Here are the steps in a PAR process, using the information in Case example 12.1.

1 Starting out—What may help prevent suicides in our community?
2 Ask the university for help in designing the research.
3 Find information from other communities.
4 Refine the question.
5 Collect some information.
6 Refine the question.
7 Collect more information.
8 Make sense of the information.
9 Check it out with community members.
10 Put it into practice—tell people about it.

Key principles of participatory action research

PAR is used in disciplines such as education, health, natural resource management, social work, and community development, and the principles for PAR apply regardless of the discipline. The key principles of PAR presented here have been adapted from Stringer (1999).

➤ The cultural values and belief systems of the host community must be understood and respected.

➤ The researchers and research participants and/or communities work together in the entire research process recognising and respecting each other's culture, expertise, knowledge and skills.

➤ The research process and the knowledge gained contributes to taking action about a real-life problem.

CASE EXAMPLE 12.2

Whether or not to continue the Internet program

A new initiative designed to provide skills for older adults in using the Internet was being trialled in a neighbourhood centre. Although the program had been widely publicised, there was a low participation rate. The neighbourhood centre staff thought it would be of value to look at why the program was not being used, whether or not it could be more relevant, or perhaps use the resources in another way. The neighbourhood centre coordinator, as a part-time student, was familiar with the research process. A PAR cycle was put in place, bringing together an advisory group of older people, some of whom had accessed the program and some who had not, neighbourhood centre staff trying to implement the program, and others who had experience in running this type of initiative. Various methods of collecting information were used. Older people interviewed people in their networks about their interest in the program, and a short press release in the local paper asked people to phone the neighbourhood to give their views. Although the PAR was time-intensive for the neighbourhood centre staff, there was a great deal of energy among participants. People enjoyed the process of asking questions about the program and trying to work out ways of finding the answers.

Think about it

➤ How does this example illustrate the principles of PAR?

➤ How is the approach useful in this situation?

➤ What are the challenges for the neighbourhood centre in using the PAR approach?

➤ The research process results in benefits to all the individuals, organisations, researchers, and communities involved.

➤ A range of information-collecting techniques can be used.

One of the crucial elements of PAR is that it involves different power relationships between the researchers and those researched than is traditionally the case. Research is portrayed as something that everyone can get involved in, and the technical words used to describe the process, such as 'methodolology', 'data', and 'analysis' are de-emphasised in favour of more user-friendly words. The term research 'subjects' is replaced by 'participants'. This helps to alter the power relationships between those with formal research expertise and those without it.

Another feature of PAR is that it seeks to change the social and personal dynamics of the research situation to enhance the lives of all who participate. It emphasises participation by people who are knowledgeable about the area of enquiry affected by it, and wish to use a research process to take action about an issue. It is a two-way education process between communities and researchers, and PAR can be used as a pathway to empower people to take action about issues. However, it is not a confrontational, or an overtly political activity. It is fundamentally a consensual approach to inquiry, and works from the assumption that cooperation and consensus-making should be the primary orientation (Stringer 1999, p. 19).

In evaluating the processes of working with communities overall, PAR is particularly useful. In health and social care development, sometimes we don't know exactly what outcomes there will be at the start of our work. While we will have clear objectives, the strategies to achieve objectives may not be apparent, and it will be through a process of planning, action and reflection that we will set indicators so that we can monitor our progress.

Designing participatory action research

There are some factors that will influence whether or not a PAR framework can be used. First, there must be a history of local involvement in service and program development, and a supportive policy context. When funding new initiatives, governments are increasingly stressing the importance of an ongoing cycle of evaluation, and it is highly likely that PAR will be an acceptable, or even a required approach. For an example of this, go to the Reconnect Program funded by the Australian Government Department of Families and Community Services (www.facs.gov.au/internet/facsinternet.nsf/via/reconnect/$file/Section6.pdf).

It is very difficult to engage in PAR research unless there are sound relationships. The community must be able to see value in contributing, and this will be more likely if communities are able to focus on a problem that they wish to solve. This does not mean that PAR research may not meet the needs of all partners. Universities frequently use a PAR design when helping communities implement new health or social care initiatives. Researchers are able to meet their own needs to research and publish through working collaboratively with communities.

Some people may find involving those who have usually been seen as 'subjects' in the research process quite challenging. However, after becoming conversant with PAR, most value the significant contributions that participants can make at all stages in the process.

CASE EXAMPLE 12.3

Creating a new employment initiative

Families in a regional centre were very interested to know more about creating employment opportunities so that young adults might have a choice of working in the community rather than going to the city. Local government was also interested in the topic as there was funding available for a new employment-creation initiative. However, the funding application had to be supported by information about the employment needs in the town. To work out how to obtain this information, local government staff called a meeting of interested residents, high school staff, and the community employment agency.

Local government personnel were clear what information was needed for the funding submission, but people at the meeting thought it would be an opportunity to ask young people, high school staff, and employers about their ideas. Young people were encouraged to get involved, and a starting point was agreed upon in the form of two research questions—what were young people's aspirations for employment in the town, and where were the employment gaps and opportunities? To obtain information for a funding submission, focused group discussions with young people were held, demographic information about the community was collected, and interviews were held with employers.

Feedback from the focus groups with young people found that the majority did not want to remain in the community when they completed high school. They were keen to look for job opportunities or attend university in the city. On the other hand, employers reported that it was difficult to get employees in the newly emerging tourism industry, and suggested that the high school should promote the industry as a career option and train students while in school. Employers suggested that the employment initiative funding could be spent on this training.

The first phase of data collected resulted in a lively debate, but no agreement about the employment needs in the town.

Think about it

➤ What do you think might have been the strengths of involving young people and employers in the research?

➤ What do you think might be the next step in the PAR cycle?

Using PAR with qualitative and quantitative methodologies

The PAR framework can include a wide variety of information-collection methods, such as interviews, focused group discussions, population surveys, literature reviews, and non-participant observation. A common mistake in thinking about PAR is to assume that only one type of research approach is possible; generally this is collecting information through a survey or a focus group. There is a tendency for surveys and focus groups to be seen as 'user friendly' and suitable to investigate community-based issues.

The PAR approach is useful as a framework within which to conduct a range of both qualitative and quantitative studies. A good example of PAR is that used by the National Aboriginal Community Controlled Health Organisation to ascertain the best method of treatment for ear infections in Aboriginal children. This was a randomised controlled trial

CASE EXAMPLE 12.4

The National Aboriginal Community Controlled Health Organisation ear trials

Couzos et al. (2005) have written about the participatory action research methods used to conduct the landmark Aboriginal community-controlled, multi-centre, double-blind, randomised, controlled clinical ear trial investigating ototopical treatments for chronic suppurative otitis media.

Evaluating community-based initiatives

The practice of evaluation has evolved with an emphasis on judgments about programs worth being undertaken by experts who are one step removed from program functioning (Johnson 2004, p. 7). In some cases, government agencies may specify an external evaluation of program. However, even in an external evaluation, community members will have knowledge about the program in its context, and can be seen as important contributors (Wadsworth 1997, p. 2).

Program evaluation is a process of assessment used to generate information about the way in which an activity is undertaken in a particular context (process) and the results of the program (outcomes). Aspects of the process and outcomes are compared against performance standards or expectations in order to make a judgment about a program's worth, merit, or value. Evaluation activities help us know more about how programs are meeting their objectives and whether or not they are relevant, accessible, and cost-effective. It is also one way to build the evidence-base about the effectiveness of particular interventions in particular contexts.

Johnson (2004, p. 3) has identified the benefits of evaluating programs:

➤ providing information to improve programs while they are ongoing;
➤ contributing to the skills development of practitioners by providing feedback on performance;
➤ contributing to best-practice standards and benchmarks;
➤ enhancing the accountability of government programs and services by providing information on performance; and
➤ helping to build the evidence-base for what types of programs work and under what circumstances.

CASE EXAMPLE 12.5

Evaluating information provision at the neighbourhood centre

A neighbourhood centre community worker had been working for more than a year to improve access to information about health and community services in an outer suburban neighbourhood. It was a diverse and rapidly growing area with new people continually moving in, and information was required about a wide range of services. Because information provision was an important part of the centre's role, the management committee decided they would find out whether or not people were getting the information they wanted. A survey was conducted at the neighbourhood centre, asking people about their enquiry, whether or not they had received appropriate information, and how the service could be improved. In addition, personnel from key health and community agencies were invited to a meeting to brainstorm the strengths and weaknesses of current practices. The agency personnel were keen to be involved as they as they valued the opportunity to hear about the practical issues that people faced in obtaining access to information about their programs. Suggestions were made about improvements that were trialled, and agency personnel met with the neighbourhood centre regularly to monitor changes.

Think about it

➤ What was the value of evaluating this program?

➤ Who were the key stakeholders?

➤ What were the benefits of engaging people from health and community agencies?

The types of evaluation

There are three types of evaluation described by Hawe et al. (1990, p. 61). These are:

➤ Process or formative evaluation, which describes and measures the activities of a program or service in its context, such as the issues in the process of establishment, whom the program is reaching, staff roles, and the governance arrangements.

➤ Impact evaluation, which describes and measures the achievement of the program objectives in the short term. For example, this may involve collecting information about what changes have been made in participants' diet at the completion of a 'healthy eating' initiative.

➤ Outcome evaluation, which describes and measures the longer-term achievements of the program. For example, one way to judge the benefits of an intensive tertiary study support program in the longer term would be to measure aspects of participants' involvement in tertiary education at six-monthly intervals after the completion of the support program.

Usually, these three types of evaluation are used in combination, and in some evaluation texts the term 'summative' evaluation is used to refer to both impact and outcome evaluation.

There are some pragmatic reasons for choosing certain types of evaluation. If, for example, a community group wants to secure refunding for a program when it has only completed its early phase, then a process evaluation is appropriate. It is not possible at this stage to answer questions about what impact that program has had on participants before they have had a chance to experience it. However, if the program has been run once, and is just about to be repeated, then both a process and an impact evaluation are possible. Participants will have views about how the program worked for them, and it will be possible to explore the achievement of objectives. Evaluating the longer-term achievements that persist over time is crucial, and can be undertaken in larger-scale projects, particularly where there is government involvement (Johnson 2004, p. 5). It is a more complex task involving considerable resources, but is most important in building an evidence-base about the effects of different types of programs (Auspos and Kubisch, 2004, p. 10).

The evaluation steps

Although there are different approaches to evaluation, the steps involved in all types are similar. The framework presented in Table 12.1 (page 254) is adapted from Johnson (2005, p. 7).

Step 1: Examining the links between program aims and strategies

The first step in the evaluation process is to examine the connections between the program aims or goals and its strategies to achieve these. The connection between goals, objectives, and strategies is known as the program logic model (Taylor-Powell et al. 1998, p. 23) or program logic (Johnson 2005, p. 8). All approaches to evaluation stress that it is at the planning stage that we think through the links between what we want to do and how we will do it, and develop the broader program objectives realistically, given the context in which we operate and the resources available (Hawe 1990). Then, having done this, we are able to identify clear performance criteria derived from the goals and objectives, and anticipated outcomes, of the program.

Identifying performance criteria at the outset is especially important in community engagement processes where the focus appears to be on undertaking community engagement because it is government policy or 'good practice' to do so, rather than on achieving specific outcomes (Johnson 2005, p. 8). Korten (1980, p. 484) critiques international aid efforts where there are many examples of contradictions between program purpose and procedure—for example, stressing

TABLE 12.1   The evaluation steps

Step 1: Examine the links between program aims and strategies ➤ Be clear about program aims and objectives ➤ Ensure that the strategies are clearly related to the aims
Step 2: Establish the purpose of the evaluation and whom to involve ➤ Decide why you want to evaluate your program ➤ Identify who are the key stakeholder groups ➤ Decide who should participate and get information from the evaluation
Step 3: Identify the key evaluation questions and information requirements ➤ Write down the evaluation questions ➤ Identify the types of information to answer the questions, including the way you will measure the program's performance
Step 4: Identify information (data) sources and collect information ➤ Find out what information already exists and how to collect it ➤ Decide what new information is needed ➤ Obtain ethics approval if necessary ➤ Develop tools to collect the information ➤ Collect the information
Step 5: Examine information and give feedback ➤ Draw conclusions from the information to answer the evaluation questions ➤ Writing reports or articles to give feedback about the evaluation ➤ Hold meetings to tell people what was learnt

participation of the poor in decision-making, but having no strategy in the project plan to facilitate people's involvement.

One of the reasons for this type of 'woolly thinking' about the connection between aims and strategies is that the program logic model was not thought through. On the other hand, sometimes there is a gap between what the funding agency requires from a program and how people would like to implement the program 'on the ground,' and the logic model reflects this. Examining the project logic model is a very important step in program planning.

Step 2: Establishing the purpose of the evaluation and whom to involve

The second step is to establish why the evaluation is to be done and who will benefit from the information obtained about the program. Evaluations may be prompted by funding agencies, by a community who wants to know whether they should support the continuation of a program, or practitioners who would like to

Activity 12.2

The New Parent program

A new program was being trialled at the community health centre. Its overall aim was to provide more effective antenatal care for new parents, mothers, and fathers. Peer support workers were to be trained and involved throughout the women's pregnancy to help deal with all the issues women were facing, including transport to ante-natal appointments, information about birthing, housing, and financial issues. However, the program did not have the resources to include fathers, and there were no objectives relating to the fathers' involvement

Think about it

➤ What are the connections between the program's aims and its strategies?

➤ What are the issues, if any, in the program logic model?

know more about the outcomes of their practice. Being clear about the purpose will determine the scale of the evaluation, and will influence the evaluation questions. Information from program evaluation can fulfil four functions:

➤ to improve program functioning;

➤ to find out what the program has achieved in the short, medium and longer term;

➤ to satisfy the organisation or the funding body that the program is worthwhile; and

➤ to establish how the program might be able to be transferred and used in other situations.

The evaluation information may be useful for practitioners, the organisation that employs the practitioners, those who receive benefits from the program, and those who sponsor it. In most cases, there are likely to be a number of different audiences, each with specific information needs. For example, the organisation that is running the program may want to evaluate the problems involved in setting up the program, and the funding body may want information about its impact. Meeting the information needs of multiple stakeholders is complex, but it is the reality within which evaluation is conducted. There are competing demands for evaluation information, and it is best to recognise and deal with these at the outset.

Wadsworth (1997, p. 12) suggests orienting the evaluation towards common ground, ensuring that the key stakeholder groups each get something from the evaluation. This can be done through establishing a 'critical reference group' to guide the evaluation. It is essential that the people who are to benefit from the program are able to effectively participate in evaluating it.

Activity 12.3

Key stakeholder groups in the New Parent program

Who do you think might want evaluation information about the New Parent program? Who are the key stakeholders?

Step 3: Identifying the key evaluation questions and information requirements

The questions that are asked to guide the evaluation are all-important. Asking questions about the process of setting up the program or service, aspects of the context that have influenced the way the program is operating, and the program's impacts and outcomes, are all relevant. But it is important only to ask questions that it is possible to answer. A frequent mistake is to ask questions about the longer-term program outcomes, when funding is only for a 'pilot' program. In this situation, it is impossible to predict whether or not the program will be operating in the longer term. This is just one of the problems with funding pilot projects, in that their value or worth is often not measured effectively.

Evaluation questions must be closely related to the program objectives, although they need not be identical. While a comprehensive evaluation will ask one or more questions related to each of the objectives, sometimes it is not feasible to do this, and there may be a focus on just one or two objectives.

Once the questions are clear, then indicators for each of the questions are developed, and these guide data collection. Indicators are the measurable aspects of the program that can tell us how the program is going. For example, an indicator that could be used in evaluating the New Parent program is the number of antenatal appointments women attended. There is a wealth of information in evaluation handbooks about the different types of indicators, process, input, output, and the use of qualitative and quantitative information. For example, see Johnson (2004).

Activity 12.4

Evaluating the New Parent program

Use the example of the New Parent program (Activity 12.5). What could be some of the questions to guide the evaluation? What information might be necessary to answer the questions?

Step 4: Identify information sources and collecting information

The process of identifying the information sources and collecting information is the stage when participants can see something happening. Collecting information that is already available, such as service usage information, minutes of meetings with details about how the program was established, or the original funding application, is the first step (Wadsworth 1997, p. 28).

Once the sources of existing information are identified, the gaps in information are apparent, and the options for obtaining new information are determined. There are a number of methods to obtain information, including:

➤ structured questionnaires;
➤ focused group discussion; and
➤ document analysis

Questionnaires

Questionnaires are useful to ask program participants and stakeholders the same set of questions in a structured manner. Respondents may answer a question by ticking a yes/no box, or saying whether they agree with statements, or they may be asked to select a response from a multiple-choice option, for example, 'Please tick the box that gives your postcode'. Some open-ended questions may be included where respondents can give their comments, for example, 'Do you have any suggestions about how the program could be improved?'

The structured questionnaire can be sent in the mail, left in waiting rooms, or people can be interviewed over the phone. The method that is used will be determined by the topic and who it is that the questionnaire is directed to. For example, if the evaluation wants to find out how much the general public knows about the program, then distributing the questionnaire widely in the community is important. If the information required is about why people don't use a particular program, then the target group will be those people who could access the program, but do not.

One of the benefits of using a structured questionnaire, compared with focus groups, is that the information to be obtained is predetermined, and decisions about how the information will be coded and used have been made. However, in some situations it may not be possible to know exactly what to ask about a program, and then a less structured approach to information-gathering may be necessary.

Focused group discussions

Focused group discussions, discussed in Chapter 11, are a way of gathering information through group discussion around set topics. Although focused group discussions are structured, they do offer opportunities to move from the set topics, if appropriate, and capture unexpected information. Focused group discussions are especially useful in obtaining the views of people with knowledge about the program, but who need the stimulation of a group discussion, or the presence of other participants, to express their ideas. With good facilitation, focused group discussion can obtain information from different perspectives and obtain a deeper understanding of some of the strengths and limitations of a program.

Running a focused group discussion needs group facilitation skills of a high order. As we discussed in the previous chapter, it is important that the facilitator be acceptable to participants and thoroughly familiar with the list of topics to be discussed. The participants need to be selected according to the type of

Activity 12.5

Collecting information about the New Parent program

You have decided that you would like to collect information from participants in the New Parent program about the usefulness of the program for them. You would also like to ask the peer support workers for their perspective, as well as the community health staff involved in establishing and maintaining the program.

Think about it

➤ What methods would you use to collect information from participants, peer support workers, and community health staff?

➤ Why have you chosen these methods?

information that is required, but also considering how participants will interact. For example, a focused group discussion on family violence may need to select participants according to age and gender.

Document analysis

Written material about the program can be collected and used in finding out about aspects of the program's functioning. It can also be used to compare with information from questionnaires and focused group discussion. The following sources of information may be relevant:

➤ published historical, sociological and demographic material about the community in which the program is operating;

➤ newspaper reports and press releases;

➤ annual reports of the sponsor of the program, minutes of meetings, and financial statements;

➤ community newsletters; and

➤ information sheets about the program.

Step 5: Examining the information and giving feedback to stakeholders

The final step in the evaluation process is to study the information collected and summarise it in relation to the questions asked in the evaluation. Does the information provide answers to the questions? What does the information show about the value or worth of the program, how it was set up, its quality, and who it is reaching? How can the information be used to inform practice, policy, and service development? Providing information about the value of the program may include its unintended consequences, how the program compares with other similar programs, and whether or not it could be used in other locations.

There are various ways to present information. Written reports often head the list, although these may be the least accessible. In addition to the report, using visual representations of the evaluation findings through making posters, diagrams, and paintings is becoming more common and in keeping with traditional Aboriginal methodologies. Often an eye-catching poster with a simple message about the evaluation findings will get the message across very effectively. Then there is presentation of information at conferences and in the media.

Practitioners and communities may be reluctant to present findings at a conference or write them up in an article. It is easy to think that 'everyone knows about this anyway—it is just common sense'. When you are close to something, it doesn't look especially novel or exciting, but viewed from the outside it can be stunning and very useful. People may not be aware of the broader audience, there may be people in another state or countries who are running a similar program and may want to access the 'common sense'.

Giving back feedback

People who have been involved in an evaluation are always curious to know the outcome, and giving the information back to participants in order that they can use it completes the evaluation cycle. It is important that this be done carefully—there should be no surprises. The crucial question is how to give feedback and whom to invite. Think about your audience and make a strategic choice rather than just 'doing the usual'.

One way to give feedback, test the relevance of the evaluation findings, and develop strategies for change is to invite key stakeholders and evaluation participants to a workshop.

If all key stakeholders are present and working together, the contributions can be invaluable in enabling research to move into action. Ensure that a succinct summary of the preliminary findings is available to all and that there is a genuine opportunity for stakeholders to comment.

Activity 12.6

Ways of giving back information about the New Parent program

One of the findings of the evaluation about the New Parent program is that the participants value having the peer support worker help with all the diverse issues they face, including some traditionally 'non-health' issues such as housing, transport, and child care. However, there are some issues with peer support workers gaining legitimacy within the health care system.

Think about it

➤ What are some creative ways to present these findings back to all the participants in the evaluation?
➤ How could the findings of the evaluation be distributed more broadly?

The evaluation timeline

It is essential to consider the timeline at the beginning of the evaluation because this may influence the methods of data collection and how much information is collected. Trying to predict how much time will be necessary to undertake the evaluation is difficult, but devising a timeline helps to ensure that the scope of the evaluation is realistic. If there is limited time in which to undertake the evaluation, it is best to adjust its scope before its commencement rather than extend the end date. Completing an evaluation timeline chart is one way to make an estimate of the time the evaluation will take.

TABLE 12.2   Evaluation timeline planner

Task	Jan	Feb	March	April	May	June
Establish evaluation reference group	■					
Develop evaluation plan	■					
Design information-collection tools		■				
Collect information			■			
Analyse information				■		
Preliminary findings					■	■
Stakeholder workshop					■	
Feedback and reporting					■	

Further information about evaluation

If people are unsure of how to go about an evaluation, then it is useful to engage with partners who have expertise, such as a university or a PHCRED program. These organisations may provide advice or be part of a critical reference group to help design the evaluation, and follow-through to help make sense of the information that has been collected.

Practice tip 12.3   Evaluation guides

There are helpful guides to assist in undertaking evaluations, including

➤ Everyday Evaluation on the Run (Wadsworth 1997)
➤ The on-line Planning and Evaluation Wizard (South Australian Community Research Unit), http://www.sachru.sa.gov.au/PEW/index.htm
➤ Evaluating Health Promotion (Hawe et al. 1990)
➤ Queensland Government Department of Communities Engaging Queenslanders: Evaluating Community Engagement (Johnson 2004)

Practice tip 12.4   Human research ethics

Approach the ethics officer at your university to check if you need ethics approved for your evaluation.

Note

1   The term 'research' is used here in its broadest sense as systematically collecting information to answer a question. Research includes evaluation as a particular type of research.

SUMMARY

This chapter stressed that research about community health and social care development is of fundamental importance in building the knowledge base to improve what we do. Increasing evidence-based practice is in focus nationally and internationally, but the processes of working with communities are complex, and there is a tendency to think that researching the work is too hard and time-consuming.

Often community work processes have complex interrelated strategies, and this is where a PAR framework is useful. The cyclical process of planning, action, and reflection enables changes to be made on the basis of the information collected.

The PAR process uses different sources of information at each step in the process, using methods to collect information such as interviews, questionnaires, focused group discussion and non-participant observation. The difference between PAR and the conventional research process is that the information gathered becomes immediately available to inform the next step in program development.

Program evaluation is the careful and rigorous process by which we establish the worth and merit of a program in the context in which it operates. A process evaluation will focus how the program was established, the contextual factors that affect the program, the program activities, and who is accessing the program. An impact evaluation measures the immediate impact of the program against its objectives, and the outcome evaluation measures the longer-term impact. Pragmatic issues, such as the resources available, and the maturity of the program at the time it is evaluated, and the resources available, will determine the type of evaluation and how much information is collected.

The steps involved in evaluating a program include clarifying the objectives of the program, determining the questions to ask, designing the tools and collecting information, analysing information and giving feedback.

USEFUL WEBSITES

Evaluation

This is the South Australian Community Health Research Unit (SACRHU) Planning and Evaluation Wizard (Murray C, Aylward P, Cooke R, Martin, M): http://www.sachru.sa.gov.au/PEW/index.htm

Tips on evaluation from the Australian government: http://www.health.gov.au/internet/wcms/publishing.nsf/Content/ruralhealth-pubs-BHC-after-learning.htm

The Australian Evaluation Society: http://www.aes.asn.au

Action research

This is a website with references to action research in many different settings: http://www.uq.net.au/action_research/arp/books.html

PHCRED

This website has information about the Department of Health and Ageing PHCRED program: http://www.phcris.org.au/phcred/index.php

The Primary Health Care Information Service—Evaluation in Primary Health Care: http://www.phcris.org.au/publications/jwatch/JournalWatch_Dec2003.pdf

Research information

The United States Department of Health and Human Services Agency for Healthcare Research and Quality has research information that is useful for communities: http://www.ahrq.gov/research/cbprrole.htm

This is a website that provides information about community-based research: http://sphcm.washington.edu/research/community.asp

ENDING UP

This chapter completes the cycle of information that has been provided about working with communities, and takes us back to the beginning. We work with communities in health and social care development in order that we can directly address inequalities in access to resources, knowledge, and opportunities to express themselves and develop. We can also address the social determinants of health that operate at the community level by working collaboratively to help build high-quality and responsive programs and initiatives.

To undertake these complex tasks, we need clarity about which community it is that we are working with. We need to know how the community functions, and whether or not there are divisions and other factors that will impact upon our work. We also need to choose an appropriate approach considering the context in which we are working and what it is we want to achieve. There are a number of useful practice frameworks that will guide us through the steps involved.

Whatever practice framework we are using, the skills involved in ensuring participative decision-making, forming and maintaining partnerships, supporting community leadership, and undertaking community planning are all essential. Each of these skill sets is involved in each of the steps. Working with communities is complex, and elements are intertwined. Currently, there is insufficient evidence to guide practice and policy, and therefore we must be open to carefully thinking about our work and take up opportunities for research and evaluation in order to improve our practice and build an evidence base. Otherwise we will never fully achieve what we set out to do—improve health and social wellbeing through working at the community level.

USEFUL WEBSITES

Evaluation

This is the South Australian Community Health Research Unit (SACRHU) Planning
       and Evaluation Wizard (Murray, C., Aylward, P., Cooke, R., Martin, M.):
       http://www.sachru.sa.gov.au/PEW/index.htm
W.K. Kellogg Foundation evaluation toolkit: http://www.wkkf.org/default.aspx?tabi
       d=75&CID=281&NID=61&LanguageID=0
The Primary Health Care Information Service—Evaluation in Primary Health Care:
       http://www.phcris.org.au/publications/jwatch/JournalWatch_Dec2003.pdf

Tips on evaluation from the Australian government: http://www.health.gov.
au/internet/wcms/publishing.nsf/Content/ruralhealth-pubs-BHC-after-
learning.htm

The Australian Evaluation Society: http://www.aes.asn.au

Action research

This is a website with references to action research in many different settings:
http://www.uq.net.au/action_research/arp/books.html

Resources for action research: http://www.emtech.net/actionresearch.htm

The United States Department of Health and Human Services Agency for
Healthcare Research and Quality has research information that is useful for
communities: http://www.ahrq.gov/research/cbprrole.htm

This is a website that provides information about community-based research:
http://sphcm.washington.edu/research/community.asp

PHCRED

This website has information about the Department of Health and Ageing PHCRED
program and the Research Capacity Building Initiative: http://www.phcris.
org.au/phcred/index.php

References

Abelson, J., Forest, P.G., Eyles, J., Smith, P., Martin, E., Guarvin, F.P. 2002, 'Obtaining public input for health-systems decision-making: Past experiences and future prospects', *Canadian Public Administration*, vol. 45, no. 1, pp. 70–97.

Abelson, J. 2001, 'Understanding the role of contextual influences on local health-care decision making: case study results from Ontario, Canada', *Social Science and Medicine*, vol. 53, no. 6, pp. 777–93.

Abelson, J., Lomas, J. 1996, 'In search of informed input: a systematic approach to involving the public in community decision-making', *Health Care Management Forum*, vol. 9, no. 4, pp. 48–51.

Alinsky, S. 1969, *Reveille for Radicals*, Vintage Books, New York.

Ansari, W.E., Phillips, C.J., Hammick, M. 2001, 'Collaboration and partnerships: developing the evidence base', *Health and Social Care in the Community*, vol. 9, no. 4, pp. 215–27.

Arnstein, S. 1969, 'A ladder of citizen participation', *Journal of American Planners*, July, pp. 216–24.

Aslin, H.J., Brown, V.A. 2004, *Towards Whole of Community Engagement: A Practical Toolkit*, Murray-Darling Basin Commission, Canberra.

Atkinson, R. 2001, 'Antenatal care and perinatal health: how to do it better in an urban Indigenous community', *Good Health—Good Country*, Proceedings of Sixth National Rural Health Conference, National Rural Health Alliance, Canberra, p. 85.

Atkinson, V., Taylor, J. 2000, 'Experiences in developing social care initiatives in regional Australia', in P. Munn & J. Farrin (eds), *Constructing Alliances Across Rural Communities*, Proceedings of the Fifth National Regional Australia Conference, Whyalla, pp. 148–56.

Auspos, P., Kubisch, A.C. 2004, *Building knowledge about community change*, The Aspen Institute, Washington.

Bagdas, B. 2005, 'Where will the next meal come from: The bread and butter issues in engagements with culturally diverse people', International Conference on Engaging Communities, Queensland Government/United Nations, Brisbane, 14–17 August 2005. <http://www.engagingcommunities2005. org/abstracts/Bagdas-Behice-final.pdf> accessed 2 September 2006.

Balloch, S., Taylor, M. (eds) 2001, Partnership Working: Policy and Practice, Policy Press, Bristol.

Bar-On, A.A., Prinsen, G. 1999, 'Planning, communities, and empowerment: An introduction to Rapid Participatory Appraisal', International Social Work, vol. 42, no. 3, pp. 277–94.

Bass, B.M. 1999, 'Two decades of research and development in transformational leadership', The European Journal of Work and Organizational Psychology, vol. 8, no. 1, pp. 9–32.

Bass, B.M., Avolio, B.J., Atwater, L. 1996, 'The transformational and transactional leadership of men and women', Applied Psychology: An International Review, vol. 45, pp. 5–34.

Baum, F. 1996, 'Community health services and managerialism', Australian Journal of Primary Health—Interchange, vol. 2, no. 4, pp. 31–41.

Baum, F., Kahssay, H.M. 1999, 'Health development structures: an untapped resource', in H.M. Kahssay & P. Oakley (eds), Community Involvement in Health Development: A Review of Concepts and Practice, World Health Organisation, Geneva, pp. 96–113.

Baum, F., Sanderson, C., Jolley, G. 1997, 'Community participation in action: an analysis of the South Australian Health and Social Welfare Councils', Health Promotion International, vol. 12, no. 2, pp. 125–34.

Bell, K., Couzos, S., Daniels, J., Hunter, P., Mayers, N., Murray, R. 2000, 'Aboriginal community controlled health services', in Department of Health and Aged Care (ed.), General Practice in Australia 2000, Commonwealth of Australia, Canberra, pp. 75–102.

Berkman, L., Glass, T. 2000, 'Social integration, social networks, social support, and health', in L. Berkman & I. Kawachi (eds), Social Epidemiology. Oxford University Press, New York.

Bernard, J.S. 1973, The Sociology of Community, Scott Foresman, Illinois.

Black, A., Hughes, P. 2001, The Identification and Analysis of Indicators of Community Strength and Outcomes, Occasional Paper No 3., Department of Family and Community Services, Canberra.

Born, P.D. 2000, Leaderful Communities: A Study in Community Leadership, unpublished Masters Thesis, Royal Roads University, Victoria, British Columbia.

Bourdieu, P. 1985, 'The forms of capital', in J.G. Richardson (ed.), *Handbook of Theory and Research for the Sociology of Education*, Greenwood, New York, pp. 241–58.

Bourke, L. 2001a, 'Rural communities', in L. Bourke & S. Lockie (eds), *Rurality Bites: The Social and Environmental Transformation of Rural Australia*, Pluto Press, Sydney, pp. 118–28.

Bourke, L. 2001b, 'One big happy family? Social problems in rural communities', in L. Bourke & S. Lockie (eds), *Rurality Bites: The Social and Environmental Transformation of Rural Australia*, Pluto Press, Sydney, pp. 89–102.

Boyce, W.F. 2002, 'Influence of health promotion bureaucracy on community participation: a Canadian case study', *Health Promotion International*, vol. 17, no. 1, pp. 61–8.

Bracht, N. (ed.) 1999, *Health Promotion at the Community Level—2—New Advances*, Sage Publications Inc., Thousand Oaks, California.

Bracht, N., Kingsbury, L., Rissel, C. 1999, 'A five-stage community organisation model for health promotion', in N. Bracht (ed.) *Health Promotion at the Community Level—2—New Advances*, Sage Publications Inc., Thousand Oaks, California, pp. 83–104.

Bramson, R.A. 2000, *Cultivating Productive Public Conversations*, Suffolk University, 2000. <http://www.prlonline.org/pdf/bramson.pdf> accessed 30 November 2006.

Brehm, J.B., Eisenhhauer, B.W., Krannich, R.S. 2004, 'Dimensions of community attachment and their relationship to well-being in the amenity-rich rural west', *Rural Sociology*, vol. 69, no. 3, pp. 405–29.

Brent, J. 2004, 'The desire for community: Illusion, confusion, and paradox', *Community Development Journal*, vol. 39, no. 3, pp. 213–23.

Bridger, J.C., Luloff, A.E. 1999, 'Toward an interactional approach to sustainable community development', *Journal of Rural Studies*, vol. 15, pp. 377–87.

Bringle, R.G., Hatcher, J. 2002, 'Campus-community partnerships: The terms of engagement', *Journal of Social Issues*, vol. 58, no. 3, pp. 503–16.

Brown, C. 1984, *The Art of Coalition Building: A Guide for Community Leaders*, American Jewish Committee, New York.

Brown, C., Lloyd, S., Murray, S.A. 2006, 'Using consecutive Rapid Participatory Appraisal studies to assess, facilitate and evaluate health and social change in community settings', *BMC Public Health*, vol. 6. <http://www.biomedcentral.com/1471–2458/6/68> accessed 13 September 2006.

Brown, I. 1994, 'Community and participation for general practice: perceptions of general practitioners and community nurses', *Social Science and Medicine*, vol. 39, pp. 335–44.

Brownlea, A. 1987, 'Participation, myths, realities and prognosis', *Social Science and Medicine*, vol. 25, no. 6, pp. 605–14.

Butler, C., Rissel, C., Khavarpour, F. 1999, 'The context for community participation in health action in Australia,' *Australian Journal of Social Issues*, vol. 34, pp. 253–65.

Butterfoss, F.D., Goodman, R.M., Wandersman, A. 1993, 'Community coalitions for prevention and health promotion', *Health Education Research*, vol. 8, no. 3, pp. 315–30.

Butterfoss, F.D., Goodman, R., Wandersman, A. 1996, 'Community coalitions for prevention and health promotion: Factors predicting satisfaction, participation, and planning', *Health Education Quarterly*, vol. 23, no. 1, pp. 65–79.

Bush, B., Dower, J., Mutch, A. 2002, *Community Capacity Index Manual*, Centre for Primary Health University of Queensland, Brisbane.

Cacioppe, R. 1998, 'An integrated model and approach for the design of effective leadership development programs', *Leadership and Organizational Development Journal*, vol. 19, no. 1, pp. 44–53.

Campbell, C., McLean, C. 2002, 'Ethnic identities, social capital and health inequalities: factors shaping African-Caribbean participation in local community networks in the UK', *Social Science and Medicine*, vol. 55, pp. 643–57.

Carroll, M.S., Higgins, L.L., Cohn, P.J., Burchfield, J. 2006, 'Community wildfire events as a source of social conflict', *Rural Sociology*, vol. 71, no. 2, pp. 261–80.

Cavaye, J. 2000, *The Role of Government in Community Capacity Building*, Department of Primary Industries, Brisbane.

Cavaye, J. 2005, 'Community engagement—new insights and learnings from practice', International Conference on Engaging Communities, Queensland Government/United Nations, Brisbane, 14–17 August 2005. <http://www.engaging communities2005.org/abstracts/Cavaye-Jim-final. pdf> accessed 29 January 2007.

Cheers, B. 1993, 'Remote region social developers', *Regional Journal of Social Issues*, no. 27, pp. 59–77.

Cheers, B. 1995, 'Integrating social and economic development in Regional Australia', Critical Social Justice Paper no. 2, Centre for Social and Welfare Research, James Cook University of North Queensland, Townsville.

Cheers, B. 1998, *Welfare Bushed: Social Care in Rural Australia*, Ashgate, Aldershot, UK.

Cheers, B. 1999, 'Rejuvenating Community in Rural Australia', in P. Munn & A. Handley (eds), *Healthy Communities for the Bush*, Proceedings of the

Third National Conference for Regional Australia and the First Broken Hill Human Services Conference, University of SA, Adelaide, pp. 2–24.

Cheers, B., Edwards, J., Graham, L. 2000, The Community Factor—A Critical Review of the Literature, unpublished working paper, Centre for Rural and Regional Development, University of South Australia, Whyalla.

Cheers, B., Luloff, A.E. 2001, 'Rural community development', in L. Bourke & S. Lockie (eds), *Rurality Bites: The Social and Environmental Transformation of Rural Australia*, Pluto Press, Sydney, pp. 129–42.

Cheers, B., Edwards, J., Graham, L. 2004, 'Community strength and health in rural communities', Proceedings of the SA PHC_RED Conference, J Fuller (ed.), Adelaide. <www.phcred-sa.org.au/ REDSnapshots2.htm> accessed 2 February 2007.

Cheers, B., Kruger, M., Trigg, H. 2005, *Community Capacity Audit Project Technical Report*, UniSA PIRSA/Rural Solutions Whyalla.

Cheers, B., Cock, G., Hylton Keele, L., Kruger, M., Trigg, H. 2005, 'Measuring community capacity: An electronic audit template', International Conference on Engaging Communities, Queensland Government/United Nations, Brisbane, 14–17 August 2005. <http://www.engagingcommunities2005. org/abstracts/S34-cheers-b.html> accessed 2 September 2006.

Cheers, B., Cock, G., Hylton Keele, L., Kruger, M., Trigg, H. 2006, 'Measuring community capacity: An electronic auditing tool', in M. Rogers & D. Jones (eds), *The Changing Nature of Australia's Country Towns*, VURRN Press, Ballarat.

Cheers, B., Darracott, R., Lonne, R. 2007, *Social Care in Rural Communities*, Federation Press, Sydney.

Chino, M., DeBruyn, L. 2006, 'Building true capacity: Indigenous models for Indigenous Communities', *American Journal of Public Health*, vol. 96, no. 4, pp. 596–9.

Cleaver, F. 2001, 'Institutions, agency and the limitations of participatory approaches to development', in B. Cooke & U. Kothari (eds), *Participation: The New Tyranny*, Zed Books, London, pp. 36–55.

Cohen, J.M., Uphoff, N.T. 1977, *Rural development participation: concepts and measures for project design, implementation and evaluation*, Rural Development Committee, Centre for International Studies, Cornell University, Ithaca, New York.

Coleman, J. 1988, 'Social capital in the creation of human capital', *American Journal of Sociology*, vol. 94, Supplement: S95–S120.

Collins, Y. 2001, 'The more things change, the more they stay the same: health care in regional Victoria', in L. Bourke & S. Lockie (eds), *Rurality Bites:*

The Social and Environmental Transformation of Rural Australia, Pluto Press, Sydney, pp. 103–17.

Commonwealth of Australia, 2001, *Better Health Care: Studies in the Successful Delivery of Primary Health Care Services for Aboriginal and Torres Strait Islander Australians*, Department of Health and Aged Care, Canberra.

Community and Cultural Services Consultancy Unit Townsville City Council, 2001, *Renewing Garbutt, People Partnerships and Planning*, Townsville City Council, Townsville.

Couzos, S., Lea, T., Murray, R., Culbong, M. 2005, 'We are not just participants—we are in change: the NACCHO ear trial and the process for Aboriginal-controlled health research', *Ethnicity and Health*, vol. 10, no. 2, pp. 91–111.

Creyton, M., See, M., Bourke P. 2005, 'Enhancing the capacity of grassroots organisations to engage: Practical initiatives from a community/local government partnership', International Conference on Engaging Communities, Queensland Government/United Nations, Brisbane, 14—17 August 2005. <http://www.engagingcommunities2005.org/abstracts/S54-creyton-m.html> accessed 2 February 2007.

Cruickshank, M., Darbyshire, A. 2005, 'Who changed Tara? A case study of community participation and engagement', International Conference on Communities, Queensland Government/United Nations, Brisbane, 14–17 August 2005. <http://www.engagingcommunities2005.org/abstracts/S89-cruickshank-m.html> accessed 2 February 2007.

de Costa, C. 2001, 'Flora's legacy', *The Lancet*, vol. 358, 2162–3.

Department of Health and Ageing 2001, *Better health care: studies in the successful delivery of primary health care services for Aboriginal and Torres Strait Islander Australians*, Commonwealth of Australia, Canberra.

Dowling, B., Powell, M., Glendinning, C. 2004, 'Conceptualising successful partnerships', *Health and Social Care in the Community*, vol. 12, no. 4, pp. 309–17.

Durie, M. 1994, *Whaiora: Maori Health Development*, Oxford University Press, London.

Dwyer, J. 1989, 'The politics of participation', *Community Health Studies*, vol. X111, no. 1, pp. 59–64.

Edmonds, L., Anglin, R. 2005, 'Community development toolkit', International Conference on Engaging Communities, Queensland Government/United Nations, Brisbane, 14–17 August, 2005. <http://www.engagingcommunities2005.org/abstracts/S117-edmonds-lf.html> accessed 2 February 2007.

Edwards, J., Cheers, B., Graham, L. 2003, 'Social change and social capital in Australia: a solution for contemporary problems'? *Health Sociology Review,* vol. 12, no. 1, pp. 68–85.

Emergency Management Australia, 2002, *Recovery, Manual 10,* Australian Government Attorney-General's Department, Canberra. <http://www.ema.gov.au/> 7 February 2007.

Eng, G., Briscoe, J., Cunningham, A. 1990, 'Participation effect from water projects on EPI (expanded projects of immunization)', *Social Science and Medicine,* vol. 30, no. 12, pp. 1349–58.

Eyre, R., Gauld, R. 2003, 'Community participation in a rural community health trust: the case of Lawrence, New Zealand', *Health Promotion International,* vol. 18, no. 3, pp. 189–97.

Fawcett, S.B., Paine-Andrews, A., Francisco, V.T., Schultz, J.A., Richter, K.P., Lewis, R.K., Williams, E.L., Harris, K.J., Berkley, J.Y., Fisher, J.L., Lopez, C.M. 1995, 'Using empowerment theory in collaborative partnerships for community health and development', *American Journal of Community Psychology,* vol. 23, no. 5, pp. 677–97.

Felton, R., Hays, T., Johnnie, H., Nallajar, S., Speechley, M., Taylor, J. 1990, 'Women Gaining Control: Self-Management in Aboriginal Women's Services', Remote Aboriginal and Torres Strait Islander Community Futures Conference, Townsville, Qld, Australian Institute of Aboriginal and Torres Strait Islander Studies.

Flora, J.L. 1998, 'Social capital and communities of place', *Rural Sociology,* vol. 63, no. 4, pp. 481–505.

Flora, J., Sharp, J., Flora, C. 1997, 'Entrepreneurial social infrastructure and locally initiated development in the nonmetropolitan United States', *The Sociological Quarterly,* vol. 38, no. 4, pp. 623–45.

Foster, G.M. 1982, 'Community development and primary health care: their conceptual similarities', *Medical Anthropology,* vol. 6, pp. 183–95.

Frankish, C.J., Kwan, B., Ratner, P.A., Higgins, J.W., Larsen, C. 2002, 'Challenges of citizen participation in regional health authorities', *Social Science and Medicine,* vol. 54, pp. 1471–80.

Franklin, M.A., White, I. 1991, 'The history and politics of Aboriginal health', in J. Reid & P. Trompf, (eds) *The Health of Aboriginal Australia.* Harcourt Brace Jovanovich Group Inc., Marrickville, NSW.

Franks, C., Curr, B., Turner, M., Poulson, K. 2007, *Keeping Company; An Intercultural Conversation,* 2nd edn, Spencer Gulf Rural Health School, Whyalla.

Freire, P. 1996, *Pedagogy of the Oppressed,* trans. M. Bergman Ramos, rev. edn, Penguin, London.

Gittell, R., Vidal, A. 1998, *Community Organising: Building Social Capital as a Developmental Strategy*, Sage, Thousand Oaks.

Goleman, D. 1998, 'What makes a leader?' *Harvard Business Review,* November December, pp. 92–102.

Gona, J.K., Hartley, S., Newton, C.R.J. 2006, 'Using participatory rural appraisal (PRA) in the identification of children with disabilities in rural Kilifi, Kenya', *Rural and Remote Health* 6: [online]. <http: rrh.deakin.edu.au> accessed 30 November 2006.

Goodman, R.M., Speers, M.A., McLeroy, K., Fawcett, S., Kegler, M., Parker, E., Smith, S.R., Sterling, T.D. Wallerstein, N.1998, 'Identifying and defining the dimensions of community capacity to provide a basis for measurement', *Health Education and Behavior*, vol. 25, no. 3, pp. 258–78.

Gore, S. 1978, 'The effects of social support in moderating the health consequences of unemployment', *Journal of Health and Social Behaviour*, vol. 19, pp. 157–65.

Granner, M.L., Sharpe, P.A. 2004, 'Evaluating community coalition characteristics and functioning: a summary of measurement tools', *Health Education Research*, vol. 19, no. 5, pp. 514–32.

Granovetter, M.S. 1973, 'The strength of weak ties', *American Journal of Sociology*, vol. 78, no. 6, pp. 1360–80.

Guterbock, T.M. 1999, 'Community of interest: Its definition, measurement, and assessment', *Sociological Practice Review*, vol. 1, no. 2, pp. 88–104.

Hancock, L. 1999, 'Health public sector restructuring and the market state', in L. Hancock (ed.) *Health Policy in the Market State*, Allen & Unwin, St Leornards, NSW, pp. 48–68.

Hartley, R. 1996, 'Leadership as a management competency in rural health organisations', *Australian Health Review,* vol. 19, no. 3, pp. 117–25.

Hasson, F., Keeney, S., McKenna, H. 2000, 'Research guidelines for the Delphi survey technique', *Journal of Advanced Nursing*, vol. 32, no. 4, pp. 1008–15.

Hassan, R. 1994, 'Temporal variations in suicide occurrence in Australia: A research note'. *Australian and New Zealand Journal of Sociology,* vol. 30, no. 2, pp. 194–202.

Hawe, P., Degeling, D., Hall, J. 1990, *Evaluating Health Promotion*, Maclennan, London.

Hawe, P., Noort, M., King, L., Lloyd, B., Jordens, C. 1997, 'Multiplying health gains: The critical role of capacity building in health promotion programs', *Health Policy*, vol. 39, pp. 29–42.

Hawe, P., Shiell A. 2000, 'Social capital and health promotion: a review', *Social Science and Medicine*, vol. 51, pp. 871–85.

Healy, K. 2006, 'Asset-based community development: Recognising and building on community strengths', in A. O'Hara & Z. Weber (eds) 2006, *Skills for Human Service Practice*, Oxford University Press, Melbourne, pp. 247–58.

Henton, D., Nguyen, C., Bramson, R.A., Bernstein, S., Gochnour, N., Hoopes, J., Lambie, J., Snyder, K., Thomas, R. 2001, *Empowering Regions: Strategies and Tools for Community Decision Making*, Monograph Series, Alliance for Regional Stewardship, Palo Alto, California. <http//www.regionalstewardship.org/Documents/Monograph2.pdf> accessed 26 May 2006.

Heller, K. 1989, 'The return to community', *American Journal of Community Psychology*, vol. 17, no. 1, pp. 1–15.

Herbert-Cheshire, L. 2000, 'Contemporary strategies for rural community development in Australia: a governmentality perspective', *Journal of Rural Studies*, vol. 16, no. 2, pp. 203–15.

Hillery, G.A. 1955, 'Definitions of community: Areas of agreement', *Rural Sociology*, vol. 20, pp. 111–23.

Hillery, G.A., 1968, *Communal Organisations: A Study of Local Societies*, The University of Chicago Press, Chicago.

Himmelman, A.T. 1992, *Communities Working Collaboratively for Change*, Humphrey Institute of Public Affairs, University of Michigan, Minneapolis.

Hord, S. 1986, 'A synthesis of research on organisational collaboration', *Educational Leadership*, February 22–26.

Ife, J., Tesoriero, F. 2006, *Community Development*, 3rd edn, Pearson Longman, Frenchs Forest NSW.

iPlan Department of Infrastructure, Planning and Natural Resources NSW. <http://203.147.162.100/pia/engagement/techniques/charette.htm> accessed 10 March 2006.

Israel, G.D., Beaulieu, L.J. 1990, 'Community Leadership', in A.E. Luloff & L.E. Swanson (eds), *American Rural Communities*, Westview Press, Boulder, Colorado, pp. 181–202.

Jacobs, B., Price, N. 2003, 'Community participation in externally funded health projects: lessons from Cambodia', *Health Policy and Planning*, vol. 18, no. 4, pp. 399–410.

Jewkes, R., Murcott, A. 1996, 'Meanings of community', *Social Science and Medicine*, vol. 43, no. 4, pp. 555–63.

Johnson, A.L. 2004, *Engaging Queenslanders: Evaluating Community Engagement*, Queensland Department of Communities, Brisbane.

Johnson, A.L. 2005, 'Evaluating community engagement: Experiences for Queensland Australia', International Conference on Engaging Communities, Queensland Government/United Nations, Brisbane, 14–17

August 2005. <http://www.engagingcommunities2005.org/abstracts/Williams-Rick-final.pdf> accessed 7 February 2007.

Johnson, D.W., Johnson F.P. 2006, *Joining Together: Group Theory and Group Skills*, 9th edn, Pearson, Boston.

Johnson P., Wistow, G., Schulz, R., Hardy, B. 2003, 'Interagency and interprofessional collaboration in community care: the interdependence of structures and values', *Journal of Interprofessional Care*, vol. 17, no. 1, pp. 69–83.

Johnson, S. 1996, 'Management of primary health care', *Australian Journal of Primary Health- Interchange*, vol. 2, no.1, pp. 98–105.

Kahssay, H.M., Oakley, P. (eds) 1999, *Community Involvement in Health Development: A Review of Concepts and Practice*, World Health Organisation, Geneva.

Kaufman, H.F. 1959, 'Toward an interactional conception of community', *Social Forces*, vol. 38, pp. 8–17.

Kawachi, I., Kennedy, B.P., Lochner, K., Prothrow-Stith D. 1997, 'Social capital, inequality, and mortality', *American Journal of Public Health*, vol. 87, pp. 1491–8.

Kawachi, I. 2001, 'Social capital for health and human development', *Health and Poverty in a Social Context,* vol. 44, no.1, pp. 31–5.

Kelly, K.J., Van Vlaenderen, H. 1996, 'Dynamics of participation in a community health project', *Social Science and Medicine*, vol. 42, no. 9, pp. 1235–46.

Kennedy, V. 2004, The Relationship Between Community Banking and Community Development in One Rural Township in New South Wales, unpublished BSW(Hons) Thesis, University of South Australia, Whyalla.

Kettner, P., Martin, L. 1986, 'Making decisions about purchase of service contracting', *Public Welfare*, Spring, pp. 30–37.

Kirk, P., Shutte, A.M. 2004, 'Community leadership development', *Community Development Journal*, vol. 39, no. 3, pp. 234–51.

Kironde, S., Kahitimbanyi, M. 2002, 'Community participation in primary health care (PHC) programmes: lessons from tuberculosis treatment delivery in South Africa', *African Health Services*, vol. 2, no. 1, pp. 16–23.

Korten, D.C. 1980, 'Community organisation and rural development: a learning process approach', *Public Administration Review*, September/October, pp. 480–511.

Kothari, U. 1999, 'Power, knowledge and social control in participatory development', in H.M. Kahssay & P. Oakley (eds), *Community Involvement in Health Development: A Review of Concepts and Practice*, World Health Organisation, Geneva, pp.139–52.

Kretzmann, J. P. 2000, 'Co-producing health: Professionals and communities build on assets', *Health Forum Journal*, January/February, p. 42.

Kretzmann, J.P., McKnight, J.L. 1993, *Building Communities from the Inside Out: A Path Toward Finding and Mobilizing Community Assets* ACTA Publications Chicago Evanston Ill. Northwestern University. <http://www.northwestern.edu/ipr/publications/community/introd-building.html> accessed 7 February 2007.

Krishna, A., Uphoff, N.T., Esman, M. (eds) 1997, *Reasons for Hope*, Kumarian Press, Connecticut.

Labonte, R., Laverack, G. 2001, 'Capacity building in health promotion, Part 1: For whom? and for what purpose?' *Critical Public Health*, vol. 11, no. 2, pp. 111–27.

Labonte, R. 1994, 'Health promotion and empowerment: Reflections on professional practice, *Health Education Quarterly*, vol. 21, no. 2, pp. 253–68.

Labonte, R. 2005, 'Community, community development and the forming of authentic partnerships, some critical reflections', in M. Minkler (ed.), *Community Organizing and Community Building for Health*, 2nd edn, Rutgers University Press, New Brunswick, pp. 82–96.

Laverack, G., Labonte, R. 2000, 'A planning framework for community empowerment goals within health promotion', *Health Policy and Planning*, vol. 15, no. 3, pp. 255–62.

Laverack, G. 2003, 'Building capable communities: experiences in a rural Fijian context', *Health Promotion International*, vol. 18, no. 2, pp. 99–106.

Legge, D., Wilson, G., Butler, P., Wright, M., McBride, T., Attewell, R. 1996, *Best Practice in Primary Health Care*, Centre for Development and Innovation in Health, Commonwealth Department of Health and Family Services, Melbourne.

Lyons, M. 2000, 'Non-profit organisations, social capital and social policy in Australia', in I. Winter, *Social Capital and Public Policy in Australia*, Australian Institute of Family Studies, Melbourne, pp. 165–92.

MacQueen, K.M., McLellan, M.A., Metzger, D.S., Kegeles, S., Strauss, R.P., Scotti, R., Blanchard, L., Trotter, R. 2001, 'What is community? An evidence-based definition for participatory public health', *American Journal of Public Health*, vol. 91 no. 12, pp. 1929–38.

Mahnken, J.E. 2001, 'Rural nursing and health care reforms: building a social health', *Rural and Remote Health* vol. 1. <http://rrh.deakin.edu.au> accessed 23 March 2002.

Martinez-Brawley, E. 2000, *Close to Home: Human Services and the Small Community*, National Association of Social Workers Press, Washington DC.

McCarthy, A., Hegney, D. 1998, 'Evidence-based practice and rural nursing: A literature review'. *Australian Journal of Rural Health,* vol. 6 pp. 96–99.

McKnight, J.L., Kretzmann, J.P. 2005, 'Mapping community capacity', in M. Minkler (ed.), *Community Organizing and Community Building for Health* 2nd edn, Rutgers University Press, New Brunswick, pp. 158–72.

McLean, S., Ebbesen, L., Green, K., Reeder, B., Butler-Jones, D., Steer, S. 2001, 'Capacity for community development: an approach to conceptualization and measurement', *Journal of the Community Development Society*, vol. 32, no. 2, pp. 252–69.

McLeay, J. 2005, (curator) *Burning Issues*, an exhibition commemorating the lower Eyre Peninsula bushfires on 11th January 2005, Graphic Print Group, Richmond, South Australia.

McMillan D., Chavis, D. 1986, 'Sense of community: A definition and theory' *Journal of Community Psychology,* vol. 14, January, pp. 6–23.

McMurray, A. 1999, *Community Health and Wellness: A Socioecological Approach*, Mosby Publishers Australia, Artarmon, NSW.

Melville, B. 1993, 'Rapid rural appraisal: Its role in health planning in developing countries', *Tropical Doctor,* vol. 23, pp. 55–8.

Midgley, J. 1986a, 'Introduction: Social Development, the State and Participation', in J Midgley, A. Hall & M. Hardiman (eds), *Community participation, social development and the state*, Methuen & Co, London, pp. i-12.

Midgley, J. 1986b, 'Community Participation: History, Concepts and Controversies', in J Midgley, A. Hall & M. Hardiman (eds), *Community Participation, Social Development and the State*, Methuen & Co, London, pp. 13–45.

Milewa, T., Valentine, J., Calnan, M. 1999, 'Community participation and citizenship in British health care planning: narratives of power and involvement in the changing welfare state', *Sociology of Health & Illness*, vol. 21, no. 4, pp. 445–65.

Minkler, M. (ed.) 2005, *Community Organizing and Community Building for Health*, 2nd edn, Rutgers University Press, New Brunswick.

Minkler, M., Wallerstein, N. 2005, 'A Health Education Perspective', in M. Minkler (ed.), *Community Organizing and Community Building for Health* 2nd edn, Rutgers University Press, New Brunswick, pp. 26–50.

Moffatt, J. 2005, 'Engaging rural and remote communities: A practice framework', International Conference on Engaging Communities, Queensland Government/United Nations, Brisbane, 14–17 August 2005. <http://www.engagingcommunities2005.org/abstracts/S71-moffatt-jj.html> accessed 2 December 2006.

Mohr, J., Spekman, R. 1994, 'Characteristics of partnership success: partnership attributes, communication behavior, and conflict resolution', *Strategic Management Journal*, vol. 15, pp. 135–52.

Mooney, G.H., Blackwell, S.H. 2004, 'Whose health service is it anyway? Community values in healthcare', *Medical Journal of Australia*, vol. 180, no. 2, pp. 76–8.

Moore, S., Sheill, A., Hawe, P., Haines, V.A. 2005, 'The privileging of communitarian ideas: Citation practices and the translation of social capital into public health research', *American Journal of Public Health*, vol. 95, no. 8, pp. 1330–7.

Morgan, L.M. 2001, 'Community participation in health: perpetual allure, persistent challenge', *Health Policy and Planning*, vol. 16, no. 3, pp. 221–30.

Moyer, A., Coristine, M., MacLean, L., Meyer, M. 1999, 'A model for building collective capacity in community-based programs: The elderly in need project', *Public Health Nursing*, Vol. 16, no. 3, pp. 205–14.

Nelson, J.O. 2001, 'Community health assessment and improvement', in R.J. Bensley & J. Brookins-Fisher (eds), *Community Health Education Methods: A Practitioner's Guide*, Boston, Jones and Bartlett, pp. 1–8.

Oakley, P., Marsden, D. 1984, *Approaches to participation in rural development*, International Labour Office, Geneva.

Oakley, P. 1989, *Community Involvement in Health Development: An Examination of the Critical Issues*, World Health Organisation, Geneva.

O'Brien, D.J., Hassinger, E.W. 1992, 'Community attachment among leaders in five rural communities', *Rural Sociology*, vol. 57, no. 4, pp. 521–34.

Ong, B.N., Humphris, G., Annett, H., Rifkin, S. 1991, 'Rapid appraisal in an urban setting, an example from the developed world', *Social Science and Medicine*, vol. 32, no. 8, pp. 909–15.

Parker, F.E., Flood K., Jarecki, S. 2005, 'Engaging farm women from culturally and linguistically diverse backgrounds in education and training', International Conference on Engaging Communities, Queensland Government/United Nations, Brisbane, 14–17 August, 2005. <http://www.engagingcommunities2005.org/abstracts /Parker-Frances-final.pdf> accessed 30 November 2006.

Parsons, T. 1951, *The Social System*, The Free Press, Glencoe, Illinois.

Patton, M.Q. 1990, *Qualitative Evaluation and Research Methods*, 2nd edn, Sage Publications Inc., Newbury Park, California.

Perlstadt, H., Jackson-Elmoore, C., Freddolino, P., Reed, C. 1998, 'An overview of citizen participation in health planning; lessons learned from the literature', *National Civic Review*, vol. 87, no. 4, pp. 347–64.

Pigg, K.E. 1999, 'Community leadership and community theory: A practical synthesis, *Journal of the Community Development Society*, vol. 30, no. 2, pp. 196–212.

Pika Wiya Health Service, Spencer Gulf Rural Health School 2004, *Gear-up Live-Longer: A Health Promotion Guide*, Pika Wiya Health Service, Port Augusta.

Poland, B., Graham, H., Walsh, E., Williams, P., Fell, L., Lum, J., Polzer, J., Syed, S., Tobin, S., Kim, G., Yardy, G. 2005, '"Working at the margins or leading from behind"?: a Canadian study of hospital-community collaboration', *Health and Social Care in the Community*, vol. 13, no. 2, pp. 125–35.

Ponce, G.A. 1995, 'Leadership does not equal what leaders do', *The Journal of Leadership Studies* vol. 2, no. 3, pp. 68–73.

Portes, A.1998, 'Social Capital: its origins and applications in modern sociology'. *Annual Review of Sociology,* vol. 24, pp. 1–24.

Putnam, R. 1993, 'The prosperous community: Social capital and public life', *The American Prospect*, vol. 13, pp. 35–42.

Putnam, R. 1995, 'Bowling alone: America's declining social capital', *Journal of Democracy*, vol. 6, pp. 65–78.

Quartermaine, L. 2003, 'What is Indigenous research'? Unpublished speech at the Indigenous Researchers Forum, Cairns.

Queensland Department of Family Services and Aboriginal and Torres Strait Islander Affairs 1994, *Remote Area Aboriginal and Torres Strait Islander Child Care Program: Services Progress Summary*, Brisbane.

Queensland Department of Family Services and Aboriginal and Torres Strait Islander Affairs 1994–1995, *Community Services Development State Plan*, Brisbane.

Queensland Domestic Violence Task Force, 1988, *Report of the Queensland Government Domestic Violence Task Force; Beyond These Walls*, Brisbane, Qld, Queensland Government Department of Family and Youth Services.

Queensland Government/United Nations International Conference on Engaging Communities, <http://www.engagingcommunities2005.org/> accessed 7 February 2007.

Rifkin, S.B. 1986, 'Lessons from community participation in health programs', *Health Policy and Planning*, vol. 13, no. 3, pp. 240–9.

Rifkin, S.B. 1996, 'Paradigms lost: Toward a new understanding of community participation in health programmes', *Acta Tropica*, vol. 61, pp. 79–92.

Rifkin, S.B., Lewando-Hundt, G., Draper, A. 2000, *Participatory Approaches in Health Planning and Promotion: A Literature Review*, Health Development Agency, London.

Rissel, C., Bracht, N. 1999, 'Assessing community needs, resources, and readiness', in N. Bracht (ed.) *Health Promotion at the Community Level—2—New Advances*, Sage Publications Inc., Thousand Oaks, California, pp. 59–69.

Robnett, B.1996, 'African-American women in the civil rights movement, 1954–1965, Gender leadership and micromobilization', *American Journal of Sociology*, vol. 101, pp. 1661–93.

Ross, S.M., Offermann, L.R.1997, 'Transformational leaders: Measurement of personality attributes and work group performance', *Personality and Social Psychology Bulletin*, vol. 23, pp. 1078–86.

Rost, J.C. 1993, 'Leadership in the new millennium', *The Journal of Leadership Studies*, vol. 1, no. 1, pp. 92–110.

Roussos, S.T., Fawcett, S.B. 2000, 'A review of collaborative partnerships as a strategy for improving community health', *American Review of Public Health*, vol. 21, pp. 369–402.

Ryan, N. 2001, 'Reconstructing citizens as consumers: implications for new modes of governance', *Australian Journal of Public Administration*, vol. 60, no. 3, pp. 104–9.

Sackett, D. 1997, 'Evidence-based medicine'. *Seminars in Perinatology*, vol. 21, pp. 3–5.

Scherer, J. 1972, *Contemporary Community: Sociological Illusion or Reality?* Tavistock, London.

Sera's Women's Shelter, 2005, *Sera's Women's Shelter, Celebrating 30 Years*, Townsville.

Sharp, J.S. 2001, 'Locating the community field: A study of inter-organizational network structure and capacity for community action', *Rural Sociology*, vol. 66, no. 3, pp. 403–24.

Shediac-Rizkallah, M.C., Bone, L.R. 1998, 'Planning for the sustainability of community-based health programs: Conceptual frameworks and future directions for research, practice and policy', *Health Education Research*, vol. 13, no. 1, pp. 87–108.

Shiffman, J. 2002, 'The construction of community participation: village family planning groups and the Indonesian state', *Social Science and Medicine*, vol. 54, no. 8, pp. 1199–214.

Short, S.D. 1989, 'Community participation or community manipulation, the Illawarra cancer appeal-a-thon', *Community Health Studies*, vol. X111, no. 1, pp. 34–8.

Smith, T.F, Fisher J., Darbas, T., Bellamy, J., Hall, l.C. 2005, 'Development of a typology of engagement in natural resource management for the western catchments of South East Queensland', International Conference on Engaging Communities, Queensland Government/United Nations,

Brisbane, 14–17 August 2005. <http://www.engagingcommunities2005.org/abstracts/S10-smith-tf.html> accessed 7 February 2007.

Sorensen, T., Epps, R. 1996, 'Leadership and local development: Dimensions of leadership in four Central Queensland towns', *Journal of Rural Studies*, vol. 12, no. 2, pp. 113–25.

Stall, S., Stoecker, R. 1998, 'Community organising or organising community? Gender and the crafts of empowerment', *Gender and Society*, vol. 12, no. 6, Special Issue: Gender and Social Movements Part 1, pp. 729–56.

Stark, A., McCullough, J.A. 2005, 'Engaging communities in community renewal, challenges, success factors and critical questions', International Conference on Engaging Communities, Queensland Government/United Nations, Brisbane, 14–17 August 2005. <http://www.engagingcommunities2005.org/abstracts/McCullough-Julie-Ann-final.pdf> accessed 7 February 2007.

Steenbergen, G., El Ansari, W. 2003, *The Power of Partnerships*, World Health Organization, Geneva.

Stone, L. 1992, 'Cultural influences in community participation in health', *Social Science and Medicine*, vol. 35, no. 3–4, pp. 409–17.

Stringer, E.T. 1999, *Action Research*, 2nd edn, Sage Publications Inc. Thousand Oaks, California.

Taylor, A., Williams, C., Dal Grande, E., Herriot, M. 2006, 'Measuring social capital in a known disadvantaged urban community: Health policy implications', *Australia and New Zealand Health Policy*, vol. 3, no. 2, pp. 2–19.

Taylor, J. 1999, 'Rural social service provision and competitive tendering against the heart', *Rural Social Work*, vol. 4, pp. 20–5.

Taylor, J., Cheers, B., Weetra, C., Gentle, I. 2004, 'Community solutions and family violence', *Australian Journal of Social Work*, vol. 57, no. 1, pp. 71–82.

Taylor, J., Fuller, J. 2004, 'Rural practitioners as researchers: The Spencer Gulf experience of research development in primary health care', *Australian Journal of Primary Health*, vol. 10, no. 1, pp.104–9.

Taylor, J. 2004, 'Community Participation in Organising Rural General Practice: Three Case Studies in South Australia', unpublished PhD Thesis, Division of Health Sciences, University of SA.

Taylor, J., Wilkinson, D., Cheers, B. 2005, 'Rural places and community participation in health services development', International Conference on Engaging Communities, Queensland Government/United Nations, Brisbane, 14—17 August 2005. <http://www.engagingcommunities2005.org/abstracts/S04-taylor-j.html> accessed 2 February 2007.

Taylor, J., Wilkinson, D., Cheers, B. 2006a, 'Is it consumer or community participation? Examining the links between "community" and "participation"', *Health Sociology Review*, vol.15, no.1, pp. 38–47.

Taylor, J., Wilkinson, D., Cheers, B. 2006b, 'Community participation in organising rural general practice: Is it sustainable? *Australian Journal of Rural Health*, vol. 14, no. 4, pp. 144–47.

Taylor, J., Edwards S., Misan G., Franks C., Angie T., Campbell S., Carlin B., Lowings C., Wanganeen R., Newchurch A., Walker J., Watkinson J. (in press), 'Effective Aboriginal community involvement in health planning: A case study', Ninth National Rural Health Conference Proceedings, Albury, 7–10 March 2007.

Taylor-Powell, E., Rossing, B., Geran, J. 1998, *Evaluating Collaboratives: Reaching the Potential*, University of Wisconsin Extension, Wisconsin. <http://cecommerce.uwex.edu/pdfs/G3658_8.PDF> accessed 7 February 2007.

Tesoriero, F. 1995, 'Community development and health promotion', in F. Baum (ed.), *Health for All: The South Australian Experience*, Wakefield Press, Kent Town, SA, pp. 268–79.

Tilley, C. 1973, 'Do communities act?' *Sociological Inquiry*, vol. 43, no. 3/4, pp. 209–40.

Towle, A., Godolphin, W., Manklow, J., Wiesinger, H. 2003, 'Patient perceptions that limit a community-based intervention to promote participation', *Patient Education and Counselling*, vol. 50, no. 3, pp. 231–3.

Trewin, D., Madden, R. 2003, *The Health and Welfare of Australian Aboriginal and Torres Strait Islander Peoples*, 4704.0, Australian Bureau of Statistics, Australian Institute of Health and Welfare, Canberra.

Turbett, C. 2006, 'Rural social work in Scotland and eastern Canada: A comparison between the experiences of practitioners in remote communities, *International Social Work*, vol. 49, no. 5, pp. 583–94.

University of Washington 2004. <http://www.fammed.washington.edu/phc/test.html> accessed 11 January 2005.

Van der Plaat, M., Barrett, G. 2005, 'Building community capacity in governance and decision-making', *Community Development Journal*, vol. 41, no. 1, pp. 25–36.

Veenstra, G. 2000, 'Social capital, SES and health: an individual-level analysis', *Social Science and Medicine,* vol. 50, pp. 619–29.

Veenstra, G., Luginaah, I., Wakefield, S., Birch, S., Eyles, J., Elliot, S. 2005, 'Who you know, where you live: Social capital, neighbourhood and health', *Social Science and Medicine*, vol. 60, pp. 2799–818.

Wadsworth, Y. 1997, *Everyday Evaluation on the Run*, 2nd edn, Allen & Unwin, St Leonards NSW.

Walter, C.L. 2005, 'Community building practice, a conceptual framework', in M. Minkler (ed.), *Community Organizing and Community Building for Health* 2nd edn, Rutgers University Press, New Brunswick, pp. 66–78.

Wandersman, A., Florin, P., Friedmann, R., Meier, R. 1987, 'Who participates and who does not and why: an analysis of voluntary organisations in the United States and Israel', *Sociological Forum*, vol. 2, no. 3, pp. 534–55.

Wandersman, A., Goodman, R.M., Butterfoss, F.D. 2005, 'Understanding coalitions and how they operate as organisations', in M. Minkler (ed.), *Community Organizing and Community Building for Health*, 2nd edn, Rutgers University Press, New Brunswick, pp. 292–313.

Warren, R.L. 1970, 'Toward a non-utopian normative model of community', *American Sociological Review*, vol. 35, April, pp. 219–28.

Warren, R.L. 1978, *The Community in America*, Rand McNally College Publishing Company, Chicago.

WHO: See World Health Organisation.

Wilkinson, D. 2000, 'Inequitable distribution of general practitioners in Australia: analysis by State and Territory using census data', *Australian Journal of Rural Health*, vol. 8, no. 2, pp. 87–93.

Wilkinson, D. 2002, 'Unhealthy encounters: Legacies and challenges for the health status of settler and Aboriginal communities', Hawke Institute, University of SA, Magill. <http://www.unisa.edu.au/ hawkeinstitute/publications/ downloads/wp17.pdf> accessed 30 January 2007.

Wilkinson, K.P. 1970, 'The community as a social field', *Social Forces*, vol. 48, pp. 311–22.

Wilkinson K.P. 1972, 'A field-theory perspective for community development research, *Rural Sociology*, vol. 37, no. 1, 43–51.

Wilkinson, K.P. 1979, 'Social well-being and community', *Journal of the Community Development Society*, vol. 10, no. 1, pp. 5–16.

Wilkinson, K.P. 1986, 'In search of the community in the changing countryside', *Rural Sociology*, vol. 5, no. 1, pp. 1–17.

Wilkinson, K.P. 1991, *The Community in Rural America*, Greenwood Press, Westport, Connecticut.

Wilkinson, K.P. 1998, 'The community its structure and process', in E. Zuber, S. Nelson & A.E. Luloff (eds), *Community: A Different Biography*, Northeast Regional Center for Rural Development, University Park PA, pp. 86–90.

Wilkinson, R. 1996, *Unhealthy Societies: The Afflictions of Inequality*, Routledge, New York.

Williams, J. 1993, 'Community services development: A new approach to government–non-government sector relations', unpublished working paper.

Williams, J. 1996, 'Policy and planning in community services—a role for government', in T. Dalton, M. Draper, W. Weeks & J. Wiseman (eds), *Making Social Policy in Australia: An Introduction*, Allen and Unwin, St Leonards, pp. 181–94.

Williams, J., Walsh, P. 1994, 'Making changes happen: The potential and challenges of collaboration in the community services industry', paper presented to the Australian and New Zealand Third Sector Conference, Negotiating the Future, July 1994.

Williams, L., Labonte, R. 2003, 'Changing health determinants through community action: power, participation and policy', *IUHPE—Promotion and Education*, vol. X, no. 2, pp. 65–71.

World Health Organisation and UNICEF 1978, *Primary Health Care: Report of the International Conference on Primary Health Care*, WHO/UNICEF, Geneva.

World Health Organisation 1986, *First International Conference on Health Promotion: Ottawa Charter for Health Promotion*, WHO, Geneva.

World Health Organisation 1991, *Community Involvement in Health Development: Challenging Health Services*, Report of a WHO Study Group, WHO, Geneva.

World Health Organisation 2000, *Primary Health Care 21: Everybody's Business: An International Meeting to Celebrate 20 Years after Alma Ata*, WHO Technical Report Series 809, WHO, Geneva.

Wright, J., Walley, J. 1998, 'Assessing health needs in developing countries', *British Medical Journal*, vol. 316, pp. 1819–23.

Yeo, M. 1993, 'Towards an ethic of empowerment for health promotion', *Health Promotion International*, vol. 8, no. 3, pp. 225–35.

Yunus, M. 1997, 'The Grameen bank story: rural credit in Bangladesh', in A. Krishna, N. Uphoff & M. Esman (eds), *Reasons for Hope*, Kumarian Press, Connecticut, pp. 9–24.

Zakus, J.D.L. 1998, 'Resource dependency and community participation in primary health care', *Social Science of Medicine*, vol. 46, no. 4–5, pp. 475–94.

Zakus, J.D.L., Lysack, C.L. 1998, 'Revisiting community participation', *Health Policy and Planning*, vol. 13, no. 1, pp. 1–12.

Zanet P., Taylor, J., Edwards, J. 2005, 'Strengthening community participation in rural communities', poster presentation, GP and PHC Research Conference, 26–28 July, Adelaide.

Index